Medical Eponyms

Diseases, Syndromes and Signs

By the same author:
(Jonathan Havard)

Blood and Judgment

The Stockholm Syndrome

Coming of Age

The Price of Fame

Published by William Heinemann Ltd.

MEDICAL EPONYMS

Diseases, Syndromes and Signs

Cyril Havard
B.Sc., M.Ch., F.R.C.S.

Barry Rose Law Publishers Ltd

© 1998 C. Havard and Barry Rose Law Publishers Ltd

ISBN 1 872328 69 5

All rights reserved. No part of this publication may be reproduced, stored in a retrieval system, or transmitted, in any form or by any means, electronic, mechanical, photocopying, recording or otherwise, without prior written permission of the authors and publishers.

Published by
Barry Rose Law Publishers Ltd.
Little London
Chichester
West Sussex

Contents

Preface	vii
Diseases	1
Syndromes	93
Signs	193
Glossary	225
References	239
Index	241

To Beth

Preface

Such is the desire for distinction amongst the medical profession that many doctors long to have some disease, syndrome or physical sign named after himself or herself. As a result, the number of eponyms is vast, a comprehensive list virtually impossible to achieve. Some eponyms are commonplace in everyday clinical practice; others describe conditions only five or six cases of which have ever been described world wide.

The final selection in a book such as this, therefore, is inevitably to some degree arbitrary.

Those chosen here are intended to be of use to all clinicians, ranging from medical students, both undergraduate and postgraduate, through established practitioners to senior consultants, faced with a strange syndrome outside his or her particular specialty. Salient features alone are given, the book designed to be a quick, table top fact finder rather than a weighty reference tome.

The medical profession is not alone in having to cope with the arcane world of eponymous nomenclature. Medical reports, required in the course of litigation, are frequently strewn with eponyms to confuse and exasperate our legal colleagues.

It is with lawyers in mind that the glossary is provided. Brief translations in lay terms are given for archaic jargon made familiar to the medical practitioner by common usage.

Liberties have been taken. Prune belly syndrome and kissing disease can hardly be called eponymous. But to have adhered strictly to the accurate interpretation would have resulted in the exclusion of several of the more important entities.

Finally, it is obvious that 300 diseases, 339 syndromes and 143 physical signs cannot be collected without widespread reference to other sources. My endebtedness to the works listed as references is gratefully acknowledged. My thanks go also to Dr John Henry Jones for his diligent proof reading.

Diseases

Addison's Anaemia
(Pernicious Anaemia.)

Megaloblastic anaemia due to failed secretion of gastric intrinsic factor.
Predominantly females.
Aged 45 to 65 years.
Increased blood destruction.
Hyperbilirubinaemia with lemon yellow skin.
Haemosiderosis.
Atrophic gastritis and sore tongue.
Subacute combined degeneration of the cord.
Macrocytosis, anisocytosis and poikilocytosis.
Nucleated red cells.
Neutropenia.
Megaloblastic marrow.
Low serum Vitamin B12.
Antibodies against gastric parietal cells.

Addison's Disease

Adrenal cortical failure.
Most commonly autoimmune disease.
Rarely tuberculous infection, amyloid infiltration, metastatic deposits, haemorrhage or infarction.
Any age; acute or chronic.
M : F :: 1 : 2.
High incidence of other autoimmune conditions.
Adrenal cortical atrophy of all three layers.
Medulla usually unaffected.
Fatigue, weakness and weight loss.
Pigmentation of the buccal mucosa and skin exposed to light or pressure.

Hypotension.
Amenorrhoea.
Acute gastro-intestinal symptoms during adrenal crisis.

Addison-Schilder's Disease

See Schilder's disease.
Schilder's disease with added involvement of peripheral nerve myelin sheaths.

Albers-Schonberg Disease
(Marble Bone Disease. Osteopetrosis.)

Congenital failure to remove bony trabeculae and replace with marrow spaces.
Bones thick and radio opaque.
Spontaneous fractures.
Cranial nerve palsies.
Hydrocephalus.
25% have leukoerythroblastic anaemia.

Albright's Hereditary Osteodystrophy
(Pseudohypoparathyroidism. Albright's Syndrome.)

Dominant hereditary abnormality of calcium metabolism.
Tetany though parathyroid function is normal.
Unresponsive to parathyroid hormone.
Pigmented skin.
Mental retardation.
Osteoporosis with bowing of long bones and fractures.
Calcium deposited in skin, brain and optic lens.

Alzheimer's Disease
(Presenile and Senile Dementia.)

Impairment of intellect, memory, emotion and behaviour.
Occurs in absence of any other cause; cerebrovascular, trauma, alcohol.
More readily recognisable in the previously intelligent, stable, meticulous.
Rate of progress varies.
Fluctuation in mood leads to total apathy.
Pathological cerebral changes include senile amyloid plaques and neurofibrillary tangles.
Typical course 5 to 10 years.

Andersen's Disease

Glycogen storage disease.
Enzyme deficiency - transglucosidase.
Failure to thrive.
Progressive hepatic cirrhosis.
Death within two years.

Aniridia-Wilms Tumour

Chromosome 11 abnormality.
Congenital partial or complete absence of the iris.
Subsequently will develop Wilms tumour.

Askin Tumour

Arises in chest wall in children.
Primitive neuroectodermal tumour.
Usually arises in rib.

Very similar to Ewing's sarcoma with similar prognosis.
Often have distant metastases at time of diagnosis.

Assman Focus

Focal lesion in adult pulmonary tuberculosis.
Almost always in lung apex.
May heal.
May cavitate.

Australia Antigen

Antigen resulting from infection with hepatitis B virus.

Baker's Cyst
(Popliteal Cyst.)

Synovial diverticulum from knee joint into popliteal fossa.
Pressure within raised during knee flexion.
Narrow neck with valvular fold preventing fluid returning to knee joint.
May rupture into calf, simulating a deep vein thrombosis.

Bankart Lesion

Detachment of the labrum and capsule from the anterior glenoidal rim.

Barlow's Disease

Impaired osteogenesis of epiphyses.
Complication of infantile scurvy.

Barrett's Oesophagus

Lower two thirds oesophagus lined with columnar epithelium.
Now considered acquired rather than congenital.
Continuous with gastric mucosa or patchy.
Cause uncertain, probably due to reflux.
Ulceration and stricture common.
10% develop carcinoma.

Bartholin Cyst

Cystic swelling in labium majus.
Blockage in duct of Bartholin's gland.
Asymptomatic if uninfected.
Liable to infection and abscess formation.

Barton's Fracture

Fracture dislocation of the wrist joint.
Distal fragment displaced anteriorly carrying carpus and hand with it.

Basedow's Disease
(v. Grave's Disease.)

Batten's Disease
(Juvenile Amaurotic Familial Idiocy.
Spielmeyer-Vogt Disease.)

Autosomal recessive metabolic enzyme disorder - chromosome 16.
Both sexes.

Diagnosed on amniocentesis.
All have progressive mental and physical deterioration.
Infantile type -
  Convulsions.
  Ataxia.
  Skull does not enlarge.
  Increasing visual loss.
Juvenile type -
  6 to 10 years.
  Loss of vision.
  Convulsions.
  Ataxia and paralysis.
  Death between 15 to 25 years.

Adult type -
  Signs begin around puberty.
  Personality changes with manic phases.
  Bursts of laughter or crying.
  Progression to severe dementia.
  Ataxia and loss of balance.
  No visual problems or convulsions.
  Survive to middle age.

Bazin's Disease

Vasculitis lower limb below knee.
Purple nodules breaking down to form indolent ulcers.
Pigmented scars.
Adolescent girls with tuberculosis.

Becker's Muscular Dystrophy

Hereditary sex linked recessive disorder.
Similar to Duchenne type.
Differs in that appears later in life and is more benign with slower progression.

Behcet's Disease

Commoner in Japan and Eastern Mediterranean countries.
Essential features -
  Aphthous stomatitis.
  Skin lesions.
  Iridocyclitis.
  Genital ulceration.
May also have -
  Large joint arthritis.
  Intestinal ulceration.
  Thrombophlebitis.
  Neuropsychiatric problems.

Bell's Palsy
(Idiopathic Facial Palsy.)

Complete facial paralysis of unknown cause.
Oedema of facial nerve in bony facial canal.
Both sexes of any age.
Eye cannot be closed.
Eye rolls upwards on attempt to close eye (Bell's phenomenon).
Paralysed side of mouth dragged over to normal side.
Dribbling saliva.
No objective sensory loss though may complain of numbness.

Occasionally oedema will involve chorda tympani with loss of taste in anterior two thirds of tongue.
90% slow recovery, only complete after 2 - 3 months.
Recurrence unusual.
May develop "crocodile tears" (weeping at meal times) owing to parasympathetic regrowth.
May develop "associated movements" (synchronous movements of eyelids and mouth) from crossed reinervation.

Bennett's Fracture

Fracture dislocation first carpo-metacarpal joint.
Inadequate reduction leads inevitably to arthritis.

Berger Disease

IgA nephropathy.
Recurrent haematuria in children.
Exacerbated by upper respiratory tract infections.

Bezold's Abscess

Complication of acute mastoiditis.
Pus breaks through the mastoid tip to form a cervical abscess.

Bietti's Nodular Dystrophy

Corneal hazing.
Common in men who have spent working life in the open air.
May progress to more severe nodular form.

Binswanger's Encephalopathy

Presenile dementia.
Result of hypertensive vascular disease.
Confined to cerebral cortex.

Bird Fancier's Lung

Allergic pulmonary reaction to organic dust.
Pigeons and budgerigars.
Cellular exudates lead to small granulomatous lesions.
Impaired pulmonary compliance, ventilation and perfusion.
Prolonged exposure produces permanent damage.

Bochdalek Hernia

Congenital absence of part of diaphragm.
Abdominal viscera herniate into chest.
90% through the Foramen of Bochdalek in posterior diaphragm.

Bockhart's Impetigo

Perifollicular staphylococcal infection.
Resembles but distinct from acne.

Bornholm Disease
(Epidemic Pleurodynia.)

Viral infection (coxsackie B) of intercostal muscles.
Severe symptoms of "dry" pleurisy.

Bourneville's Disease
(Tuberous Sclerosis. Pringle Disease.)

Inherited as dominant trait but not always penetrant.
Epilepsy.
Mental deficiency.
Nodular facial rash (adenoma sebaceum).
C.T. brain scan shows calcified masses (tubers).

Bowen's Disease
(Carcinoma in Situ.)

The presence of tumour cells in the skin; intra-epidermal carcinoma.
Limited to epidermis with intact basal membrane.
Appearances and staining characteristics of malignancy but non-invasive.
Histologically characteristic Bowen cells have large, hyperchromatic nuclei with vacuoles giving haloed appearance.
Commonest on trunk, hands and feet.
Also in perianal and genital areas.
Analagous to changes in uterine cervix, prostate, penis and Paget's disease of nipple.

Brenner Tumour

Hard solid ovarian tumour.
Composed of transitional or squamous epithelium in dense fibrous stroma.
Usually benign.

Bright's Disease
(Glomerulonephritis.)

Acute, subacute and chronic stages.
Acute nephritic stage -
   Immune reaction; may follow beta-haemolytic streptococcal throat infection.
   Haematuria.
   Oliguria.
   Hypertension.
   Uraemia.
   Periorbital oedema.
Subacute nephrotic stage -
   Swollen, smooth, pale kidneys.
   Generalised oedema.
   Proteinuria.
   Hypoproteinaemia.
Chronic stage -
   May give no history of acute or subacute stages.
   Small scarred kidneys.
   Uraemia.
   Renal failure.
   Fibrosis of glomeruli and fibrous replacement of tubules.

Brill's Disease

Mild relapse after typhus attack.
May occur many years after initial attack.

Brodie's Abscess

Indolent bone infection.
History of preceding acute infection may be absent.

Usually result of delayed or inadequate treatment of osteomyelitis.
Circumscribed cavity with dense walls.
Sequestrum formation.
Usually requires surgical drainage and sequestrectomy.

Brodie's Serocystic Sarcoma

Rapidly growing tumour of breast.
Usually young girls after puberty.
Usually benign but may appear malignant due to rapid growth.

Bruns Frontal Ataxia

Impaired gait with small steps.
Sign of frontal cerebral lesion.

Bruton's Agammaglobulinaemia

Sex linked - boys only.
Apperas about six months as maternal immunity is exhausted.
Absent Payer's patches, tonsils and appendix.
Absence of immunoglobulins.
Absence of plasma cells from lymph nodes.
Absence of circulating B lympthocytes.
Arthropathies.
Susceptible to severe infections.

Buerger's Disease
(Thromboangiitis Obliterans.)

Men before age of 40.
Heavy smokers.

Mainly affects lower limbs.
Thrombosis in artery with artery wall infiltrated with lymphocytes.
Recurrent phlebitis (thrombophlebitis migrans) may also occur.
Intermittent claudication and rest pain.
Ischaemia leading to gangrene.

Burkitt's Tumour
(African Lymphoma.)

Non-Hodgkin lymphoma.
Endemic in regions with temperature range above 60° F and rainfall over 20 ins.
Similar endemic distribution to that of trypanosomiasis.
Suggests a carcinogenic viral infection (Epstein-Barr) via insects.
E-B viral antibody found in most cases.
Children 3 - 9 years old.
Arises in predominantly extranodal tissue; jaws, kidneys, ovaries, heart and paravertebral regions.
Orbital deposits extrude the eye.
Primitive lymphoid cells with clear histiocytes giving "starry sky" appearance histologically.
Metastasises widely with paraplegia from spinal extradural deposits.

Buruli Ulcer

Caused by mycobacterium ulcerans.
Chronic ulcer commonly on limbs.
Necrosis of subcutaneous nodule.
Spreads laterally.
Overhanging edge to ulcer.

Begins to heal after several weeks.
Healing may take years.

Buschke-Loewenstein Tumours
(Condylomata Acuminata.)

Genital warts of extreme size.
Usually on prepuce.

Caffey's Disease
(Caffey's Syndrome. Infantile Cortical Hyperostosis.)

Hereditary disorder of periosteum and cortical bone.
Infants less than six months old.
Malaise, fever and painful swelling of long bones, mandible and scapula.
Easily mistaken for osteomyelitis.
Exacerbations with fever and irritability.
Penicillin therapy very successful.
Capable of spontaneous resolution.

Caisson Disease
(Decompression Sickness. The Bends.)

Too rapid return from high pressure to atmospheric.
Too rapid change from atmospheric to low pressure.
Air bubbles come out of circulating blood.
Oxygen and carbon dioxide are rapidly absorbed.
Inert nitrogen remains.
Results in mechanical tissue damage, particularly neural.
Severe pain (the bends).
Bubbles in extradural venous complex obstructs venous return from cord.

Sometimes permanent paraplegia or death.

Camurati's Disease
(v. Engelmann's Syndrome.)

Canavan's Disease
(Spongiform Leucodystrophy.)

Inherited disorder of myelin metabolism (leucodystrophy).
Common in Ashkenasi Jews.
Presents at three months of age.
Spasticity and enlarging head.
Aphasia.
Seizures.
Ataxia.
Dementia.
Optic atrophy and blindness.
Usually fatal before three years of age.

Caroli's Disease

Hereditary autosomal recessive.
Multiple intrahepatic cysts.
Recurrent cholangitis.
Intrahepatic calculi.
Liver abscesses.
Cirrhosis.
Poor prognosis.

Carrion's Disease
(Bartonellosis. Oroya Fever.)

Infection by Bartonella bacilliformis.
Transmitted by sandflies.
South American countries.
Endemic in Andean region of South America.
Invades and destroys red cells.
Severe haemolytic anaemia.
Muscle and joint pains.
Diarrhoea and vomiting.
Delirium and coma.
Haemoptysis.
Early treatment gives good results.
Untreated - 90% mortality.

Carr's Concretions

Microconcretions within kidney substance.
Thought due to lymphatic obstruction.
May ulcerate into collecting tubules.

Ceelen's Disease
(Idiopathic Pulmonary Haemosiderosis.)

Possibly auto-immune.
Brown induration of the lungs.
Previously healthy young children.
Diffuse intra-alveolar haemorrhages throughout lungs.
Pallor, dyspnoea, cyanosis, fever and tachycardia.
Hepatosplenomegaly.
Cardiomegaly, gallop rhythm and cardiac failure.
Jaundice may occur.

Chagas' Disease
(American Trypanosomiasis.)

Infection with Trypanosoma Cruzi.
South and Central America.
Transmitted via skin contamination with faeces of reduviid bug.
Entry through conjunctiva (Romana's sign), oral mucosa or abrasion.
Form pseudocysts in myocardium and autonomic ganglion cells.
Fever and lymphadenopathy.
Hepatosplenomegaly.
Damage to Auerbach's plexus causes bowel dilatation, especially colon and oesophagus.
Occasionally mimics achalasia of the cardia.
Cardiomyopathy gives arrhythmias, heart block and sudden death.

Charcot's Fever
(Charcot's Triad.)

Epigastric pain.
Rigors.
Jaundice.
Caused by ascending cholangitis.
May be fatal especially in elderly when jaundice may not be obvious.
May present simply as shock due to septicaemia.

Charcot's Joints
(Neuropathic Joints.)

Painless, swollen, unstable joints in sensory neurological disorders.
Usually large joints - hip, knee, ankle.

Tabes dorsalis.
Syringomyelia (upper limbs).
Diabetic neuropathy.

Chikungunya Fever

Arboviral infection (i.e. arthropod borne).
Transmitted by mosquito (Aedes aegypti).
Haemorrhagic fever of Africa.
Fever with maculopapular rash.
Photophobia and pain in orbit.
Arthralgia and myalgia, often severe.
May develop encephalitis, haemorrhage and circulatory failure.

Chimney Sweep's Cancer

Epithelioma of scrotum.
First occupational cancer to be documented (Percival Pott 1775).
Chemical carcinogens in soot and coal tar.

Christensen-Krabbe Disease
(v. Alpers Syndrome.)

Christmas Disease
(Haemophilia B.)

X linked recessive bleeding disorder.
Linked to deficiency of factor 9.
Males only.
Female carriers transmitting to 50% of male children.
Bruising.

Haemarthrosis.
Degree of severity depends on degree of factor deficiency.
High incidence of iatrogenic hepatitis B infection.

Clark's Naevus
(Atypical Naevus. B-K Mole.)

Dysplastic naevus occurring in melanoma prone families.
May occur in up to half family members.
Vary in colour, shape size, number and location from benign acquired naevi.

Clay Shoveller's Disease

Avulsion fracture spinous process seventh cervical vertebra.

Clutton's Joints

Painless effusion into the knee joints in adolescents.
Syphilitic in origin.
Now rarely seen.

Coat's Disease

Most severe form of retinal telangiectasis.
Always unilateral.
Commoner in boys.
Usually first decade.
Strabismus.
Visual loss.

Cock's Peculiar Tumour

Infected sebaceous cyst.
Usually on scalp.

Colles Fracture

Fracture at the wrist.
Common in elderly with osteoporosis.
Lower end of radius displaced backwards and tilted both backwards and sideways (radially).
Ulnar styloid usually avulsed.
Typical "dinner fork" deformity.

Cooley's Anaemia
(Beta Thalassaemia.)

One of heterogenous group of disorders of haemoglobin synthesis.
Suppression of beta chain formation.
Chronic haemolytic anaemia.
Appears in infancy, not newborn.
Pallor.
May be jaundiced.
Hepatosplenomegaly.
Diabetes mellitus and other endocrine disorders.
Skeletal changes - radiologically skull shows "hair on end" appearance.
Mongoloid facies and broad hands.
"Target cells" are seen in blood.
Growth retardation.
Most die in adolescence due to cardiac failure due to iron overload.

Cori's Disease

Autosomal recessive.
Children with glycogen storage failure.
Enzyme deficiency - glucosidase
Accumulation of abnormal glycogen.
Splenomegaly.
Hepatomegaly tending to diminish at puberty.
Gout does not develop.
Resembles milder form of von Gierke's disease.

Creutzfeldt-Jakob Disease

Subacute spongiform encephalopathy.
Presenile dementia.
Epilepsy and stupor.
Myoclonus and ataxia.
Motor neurone disorders.
Death in a few months.
Caused by prion similar to that found in BSE (Bovine Spongiform Encephalopathy) and scrapie in sheep.

Crohn's Disease

Non specific granulomatous bowel disease.
Histologically resembles tuberculosis or sarcoid but no caseation.
Most commonly found in terminal ileum.
May also occur in "skip lesions" anywhere from mouth to anus.
Adolescence or early adult life.
Rarely acute onset.
Usually chronic and insidious with colic, diarrhoea and general malaise.

Subacute obstruction.
Typical Kantor's "string sign" in terminal ileum on barium studies.
Mucosa shows "cobble stone" pattern with linear ulceration.
Perforation rare.
Localised abscess and fistula formation .
Recurrent perianal infections.
Polyarthritis and iridocyclitis.

Curling's Ulcer

Acute peptic ulceration in cases of severe burns.
Originally described as duodenal ulcer in children.
May occur at any age.
Gastric erosions may be multiple.
May bleed but perforation is rare.
May also occur with intracranial trauma and tumour.
These latter differ from burns as they are deep and may perforate.

Cushing's Disease

Due specifically to adrenal cortical hyperplasia under influence of pituitary.
All the features of Cushing's syndrome.
M : F :: 1 : 4.
Obesity with purple striae and "buffalo hump".
Muscle wasting.
Florid appearance with "moon" face.
Hypertension.
Skin atrophy with haemorrhages.
Osteoporosis.
Diabetes mellitus.

Suppressed ovulation with amenorrhoea.
Hirsutism and acne.
Remission of symptoms is possible if cause of excess cortisol production is removed.
Structural changes to heart, blood vessels, kidneys and bone likely to remain.

Cushing's Ulcer

In oesophagus, stomach and duodenum.
Occur with intracranial tumour or trauma or after craniotomy.
Deep and penetrating.
Tendency to necrosis and perforation.

Dejerine-Sottas Disease

Hereditary recessive.
Onset in infancy.
Neuropathy with palpable nerve trunks.
Very slow conduction velocity.
Severe weakness.
Sensory ataxia.
Areflexia.
Absent tendon jerks.
Marked rise in CSF protein.

Dejerine-Thomas Disease

Dysarthria.
Urinary incontinence.
Impotence.
Generalised myoclonus at rest.

Muscular rigidity.
Due to ponto-cerebellar atrophy.

de Quervain's Disease
(Subacute Thyroiditis.)

Usually women between 40 to 50 years of age.
Usually follows a viral (coxsackie B) or upper respiratory infection.
Thyroid swollen, firm and tender.
Thyroid function suppressed.
Raised sedimentation rate.
Histology shows infiltration with mononuclear and giant cells.
Usually recovers spontaneously.
Subsequent hypothyroidism rare.
Surgery seldom indicated.

de Quervain's Tenosynovitis

Tenosynovitis where tendons of extensor pollicis brevis and abductor pollicis longus pass through groove on lower end of radius.
Pain base of thumb.
Pain worse on abducting thumb against resistance.
Pain worse on passively abducting thumb across the palm.
Tenderness localised over radial styloid.
May have palpable or audible crepitus.
Usually result of repetitive strain.

Dercum's Disease
(Adiposis Dolorosa.)

Subcutaneous lipomatosis.

Deposits may be extreme.
Painful to touch.

Devic's Disease
(Neuromyelitis Optica.)

Common in Japanese men.
Sudden transverse cord lesion.
Bilateral demyelinating optic neuritis.
May be presenting symptoms of multiple sclerosis.
May occur in Behcet's syndrome or systemic lupus erythematosus.

Dhobi itch
(Tinea Cruris.)

Ringworm infection of groin.
Often associated with infection on feet.

Dietl's Crisis

Loin pain.
Nausea and vomiting.
Tachycardia and hypotension.
Caused by ureteric obstruction.

Di Guglielmo's Disease
(Acute Erythraemic Myelosis.)

Neoplastic condition of the erythrocyte.
Results in a form of erythroblastic leukaemia.

Red cells in all stages of maturity.
Erythroid infiltration of liver and spleen.
Bone marrow full of every erythropoietic element.
Clinical course indistinguishable from acute myeloid leukaemia.

Duchenne Muscular Dystrophy
(Progressive Pseudo Hypertrophic Muscular Dystrophy.)

X linked recessive enzyme disorder.
Males only.
Female carriers.
Though X linked, half affected boys are isolated cases from mutant carriers.
Genetic counselling important.
Symptoms appear in first five years.
Delayed walking.
Lumbar lordosis and waddling gait.
Loss of balance.
Rises from a fall by "walking" his hands up his legs to the upright position (Gower sign).
Enlarged (pseudohypertrophy) of leg muscles due to fibro-fatty infiltration.
Chest deformities with breathing difficulties.
Heart muscle also affected with congestive cardiac failure.
Intellectually normal but wheelchair by 8 to 11 years.
Death from respiratory failure in late teens.
Serum enzyme changes (high level of creatine phosphokinase) may precede clinical manifestation and may be used to detect female carriers.
Diagnosis confirmed by electromyograph and muscle biopsy.

Duhring's Disease
(Dermatitis Herpetiformis.)

Chronic vesicular skin disease.
Forearms, scapular and sacral areas, buttocks and thighs.
2/3 have enteropathy similar to coeliac disease.

Dupuytren's Contracture

Acellular fibrous thickening of palmar aponeurosis in elderly men.
Adheres to overlying skin.
Often bilateral.
Causes flexion deformities at metacarpophalangeal and proximal interphalangeal joints.
Ring finger worst affected.
Mendelian dominant.
Progresses slowly in the elderly.
More aggressive in younger age groups.

Eales Disease

Recurrent retinal and vitreous haemorrhages.
Both eyes.
Usually young adult males.
Sudden blurring of vision.
Unknown aetiology.

Eck Fistula

Anastomosis of portal vein to inferior vena cava.
Bypasses liver in treatment of portal hypertension.

Eight Day Disease
(Neonatal Tetanus.)

Failure to suckle on third day.
Facial spasms (risus sardonicus) on eighth day.
Spasm of masseter (lock jaw).
Generalised clonic spasms.
Flexed arms with clenched fists.
Extended legs with plantar flexed toes.

Epstein-Barr Virus

Herpes virus first isolated from Burkitt's tumour.
Found in cell cultures from patients with infectious mononucleosis.
May play part in aetiology of nasopharyngeal malignancy.
Associated with the lymphoma occurring in transplant patients on long term immunosuppression.

Erb's Muscular Dystrophy
(Juvenile Scapulo-humeral Muscular Dystrophy.)

Autosomal recessive muscle disorder.
Nervous system not involved.
Both sexes.
Usually 10 to 30 years old.
Starts in one shoulder and spreads to both.
May affect pelvic girdle.
Progressive, symmetrical wasting and weakness.
Rarely survive to middle age.
Confirmed by electromyography or muscle biopsy.
Serum enzyme changes may precede clinical manifestations.

Erb's Palsy
(Erb-Duchenne Paralysis.)

Stretching of upper brachial plexus.
Most commonly after manipulation during breech presentation.
Paralysis of abduction at the shoulder, flexion at the elbow, supination and extension at the wrist.
Arm becomes adducted, extended at elbow, internally rotated with flexed, pronated wrist; the "waiter's tip" position.
Usually resolves spontaneously.

Erdheim's Cystic Medionecrosis

Myxomatous change in aortic wall.
Degeneration of elastic fibres results in aneurysmal dilatation and dissecting aneurysm seen in Marfan's syndrome.

Ewing's Tumour
(Ewing's Sarcoma.)

Usually mid shaft of long bone.
May be multicentric.
Up to 25% of all malignant chest wall tumours.
"Onion skin" layers of bone.
Not osteogenic.
Histologically - sheets of small round or polyhedral cells with little or no intercellular substance (c.f. osteogenic sarcoma).
Many now considered to be primitive neuroectodermal in origin.
May spread to lymph glands as well as lungs.
Very radiosensitive.
Fever.
Anaemia.

Swelling.
Pathological fractures.

Fabry Disease
(Fabry-Anderson Disease.
Angiokeratoma Corporis Diffusum.)

X linked recessive enzyme disorder.
Predominantly males.
Excessive lipid deposits in blood vessels.
First symptoms in childhood.
Pain in fingers and toes, later in arms and legs.
Attack may last weeks.
Triggered by tiredness or sudden change in environmental temperature.
Skin angiokeratomata.
Corneal opacities.
Renal failure after age 10.
Coronary heart disease.

Fallot's Tetralogy

Pulmonary stenosis (atresia in most severe cases).
Ventricular septal defect.
Aorta displaced to right to override the septum.
Right ventricular hypertrophy.
Other anomalies may co-exist.
Pulmonary oligaemia.
Central cyanosis after ductus closes due to diversion of unaerated blood from right to left.
Blue baby.
Dyspnoea; squats at play.

Weak and stunted with finger clubbing.
Polycythaemia with pulmonary and cerebral thrombosis.

Fanconi Anaemia

A chromosome instability syndrome.
Typically presents 4 to 6 years old.
Hypoplastic anaemia.
Pancytopenia.
Splenic hypoplasia.
Multiple congenital abnormalities of skeleton and central nervous system.
Abnormality in DNA repair leads to increased tendency to leukaemia and lymphoma.
50% have skin pigmentation.

Farmer's Lung

Allergic pulmonary reaction to organic dust.
Micropolyspora faeni in mouldy hay.
Cellular exudates lead to small granulomatous lesions.
Impaired pulmonary compliance, ventilation and perfusion.
Prolonged exposure produces permanent damage.

Fordyce's Disease

Clusters of yellowish masses in oral mucosa due to aberrant sebaceous glands.

Forestier's Disease
(Ankylosing Hyperostosis.)

Fairly common in older men.
Widespread ossification in spinal ligaments and tendons.
Changes in spine simulate ankylosing spondylitis.
Sacro-iliac joints spared.
ESR normal.

Fournier's Gangrene

Gangrene of scrotum.
Haemolytic streptococcal infection.
May be spontaneous.
Usually follows trauma or operation.
Does not involve testis.
May spread on to abdominal wall.
May involve considerable skin loss.

Freiburg's disease

Osteochondritis head of either second or third metatarsal.
Adolescence.
Pain base of toe and sole of foot.

Friedreich's Ataxia

Hereditary autosomal recessive disorder of chromosome 9.
Spinal cord atrophy in both sexes.
Normal up to age 3 years.
Symptoms may be delayed until puberty.
Ataxia, beginning in legs, with broad based, lurching gait.

Arms involved later.
Weakness and proprioceptive sensory loss.
Sense of touch lost; pain and temperature intact.
Scoliosis and high arched feet.
Most are confined to wheelchair by 25 years.
Nystagmus and occasional deafness.
Cardiomegaly with dyspnoea and palpitations.
20% become diabetic.

Galeazzi Fracture

Fracture shaft of radius with subluxation at distal radio-ulnar joint.
Ulna is intact.

Gamstorp's Disease
(Adynamia Episodica Hereditaria.)

5 to 15 years old.
Sudden onset weakness 30 minutes after exercise.
May delay further attack by more exercise.
Delayed attack thereby made more severe.
Proximal muscles.
May remit after 20 years.

Garre's Disease
(Non Suppurative Osteomyelitis. Sclerosing Osteomyelitis.)

Adolescent or young adult.
Low grade pain and bony swelling.
No abscess cavity.
Diffuse area of bony sclerosis.
May mimic Ewing's sarcoma.

Gartner's Cyst

Cystic remnants of mesonephric ducts in the female.
May occur adjacent to Fallopian tube, anterolateral border of uterus or upper vagina.
Usually symptomless.

Gaucher's Disease

Autosomal recessive enzyme (glucocerebosidase) disorder.
Likely to be in Ashkenazy Jew.
Results in lipid accumulation.
Generalised haemosiderosis with brown skin pigmentation.
Pingueculae (pigmented scleral thickenings).
Characteristic Gaucher cells appear in marrow.
Two types; neuropathic and visceral.
Neuropathic presents in infancy -
  feeding problems,
  stridor,
  spasticity,
  mental retardation,
  death from respiratory failure before 2 years.
Visceral presents in childhood or early adulthood -
  hepatosplenomegaly,
  anaemia,
  yellow skin,
  bone erosion with pathological fractures but reasonable life span.

Ghon Focus

Primary lesion in pulmonary tuberculosis.
Usually children.

Parenchymal nodule with enlarged regional hilar glands.
Often becomes calcified.

Glanzmann's Thrombasthenia

Inherited autosomal recessive platelet functional disorder.
Due to deficiency of glycoproteins.
Defect is in platelet function, not numbers.
Bleeding time prolonged.
Mild bleeding tendency due to abnormal clot retraction and defective platelet aggregation.
Epistaxis, bleeding gums, menorrhagia, ecchymoses.
Post trauma bleeding may be severe.

Gorham's Disease

Massive osteolysis.
Associated with haemangiomata and lymphangiectasis.
May present with pathological fracture.
Usually contiguous bones but may present in multiple sites.

Grave's Disease
(Primary Thyrotoxicosis. Basedow's Disease. Parry's Disease.)

Autoimmune hyperthyroidism.
M : F :: 1 : 7.
Overactivity in a diffusely enlarged thyroid, c.f. Plummer's disease.
Smooth uniform goitre with bruit, sometimes palpable thrill.
Increase in metabolic rate.
Tremor, anxiety and emotional instability.

Intolerance to heat.
Weight loss with increased appetite.
Sinus tachycardia.
Auricular fibrillation particularly in the elderly.
Warm, moist skin with capillary pulsation.
Exophthalmos, occasionally "malignant".
Eye signs; lid lag, lid retraction, difficulty in convergence.
Pretibial myxoedema in severe cases.
Muscle weakness (thyrotoxic myopathy).
Histologically vascular with small, empty thyroid vesicles with tall epithelium.

Grawitz Tumour
(Hypernephroma.)

Painless haematuria.
Loin pain.
Abdominal mass.
May present with metastasis; spontaneous fracture, paraplegia.
Lung metastases may rarely regress spontaneously after nephrectomy.

Gritti-Stokes Amputation

Through knee amputation.
Patella is fixed over cut end of femur.
Well vascularised anterior flap.
Partially end weight bearing stump.

Grumbach's Disease

Congenital hepatic fibrosis.
Multiple intrahepatic cysts (see Caroli's disease).

Hallevorden-Spatz Disease

Degenerative disease of children.
Progressive dystonia.
Hyperkinesia.
Retinitis pigmentosa.
Mental deterioration.

Hand-Schuller-Christian Disease

Eosinophilic granuloma of bone.
Mainly 5 to 10 year old.
Well demarkated lytic lesions.
Most commonly skull, ribs, clavicle and vertebrae.
Painful swellings.
Occasional spinal cord compression.
Deposit in mastoid with persistent ear discharge.
Skin rash.
Exophthalmos.
Diabetes insipidus.
Hepatosplenomegaly.
Cystic lung and spontaneous pneumothorax.
Spontaneous remission possible.

Hangman's Fracture

Bipedicular neural arch fracture of C2 (axis) vertebra.
Over 10% of all cervical spine injuries.

Hanot's Cirrhosis
(Primary Biliary Cirrhosis.)

Aetiology uncertain.

Predominantly middle aged women.
Afebrile.
No evidence of infection.
Obstructive jaundice with normal biliary tree.
Skin also pigmented.
May survive for many years.
Portal hypertension and liver failure in terminal stages.

Hansen's Disease

Leprosy; infection with Mycobacterium leprae.
Infection probably by inhalation during childhood.
Resistance to culture in vitro makes pathological diagnosis difficult.
Attacks skin, nerves and upper respiratory mucosa.
First scaly skin patch (indeterminate lesion) may heal spontaneously.
Dermis packed with macrophages (lepra cells) lead to ulcerating skin lesions.
Leonine facies with destruction of nasal bones.
Gross deformities due to sensory loss and paralytic contractures.

Hartnup Disease

Autosomal recessive metabolic disorder.
Impaired absorption of tryptophan causing Vitamin B (nicotinic acid) deficiency
Pellagrous dermatitis.
Behavioural abnormalities.
Neuropathies including episodic cerebellar ataxia.
Hyperreflexia.
Respond to nicotinamide.

Hashimoto's Disease
(Lymphadenoid Goitre.)

Autoimmune disease of thyroid.
Predominantly middle aged female.
M : F :: 1 : 15.
May occur in normal thyroid or in pre-existing goitre.
Aching pain and slight dysphagia.
Thyroid enlarged and firm.
Histologically widespread lymphocytic infiltration of thyroid.
Rarely invades overlying strap muscles.
High thyroglobulin titre.
Mild hypothyroidism but rarely hyperthyroid (Hashitoxicosis).
Microscopy shows parenchymal atrophy with diffuse fibrosis and lymphocyte infiltration.

Henoch Schonlein Purpura

Especially in children.
Anaphylactoid form of purpura.
Acute vasculitis affecting arterioles and venules.
Life rarely threatened from blood loss.
Non-thrombocytopenic.
Abdominal pain and vomiting
Localised oedema face, hands, feet and scrotum.
Acute arthritis of one or two joints at a time.
Maculopapular rash buttocks and extensor surfaces of limbs.
Mild focal glomerulonephritis.
Self limiting, lasting less than three months.
More serious cases may have intussusception, rectal bleeding or haematuria.
Renal damage may be only permanent effect.
Responsible for 5% of children requiring renal dialysis.

Hers's Disease

Glycogen storage disorder.
Heterogeneous group of mild forms of von Gierke's disease.

Hirschprung's Disease

Commoner in boys.
Functional disorder of pelvirectal junction.
Failure of neural crest cells migration to gut.
Results in congenital loss of parasympathetic nerve supply.
Biopsy reveals absence of ganglion cells and parasympathetic nerve fibres from local myenteric plexus.
Bowel fails to dilate ahead of wave of contraction.
Colon above becomes grossly distended and hypertrophied.
Bowel below appears normal and empty.
Constipated from birth.
Gross abdominal distension.

Hodgkin's Lymphoma

Painless enlargement lymphoid tissue.
Any age in both sexes.
Usually lymph nodes.
Normal histological architecture destroyed by proliferating lymphoid cells.
Differentiated from non-Hodgkin lymphoma by presence of Reed-Sternberg cells.
Predominant cell will determine degree of aggression.
Hepatosplenomegaly.
Bone marrow, lungs and kidneys may also be affected.
Discrete, mobile glands may cause obstructive symptoms.

Fever (Pel Ebstein) and night sweats.
Generalised pruritis.
Pain in glands on drinking alcohol.
Progressive haemolytic anaemia.
Leucocytosis and lymphopenia.
Diagnosis by lymph node biopsy.
Potentially curable.

Humidifier Lung

Reaction to antigen from thermophilic bacteria in air conditioning systems.
May produce chronic, progressive pulmonary disease.

Hunner's Ulcer
(Interstitial Cystitis.)

M : F :: 1 : 10
Stellate ulcers on bladder vault.
Grossly reduced bladder capacity.
Severe frequency and urgency.
Urine sterile.
May be associated with autoimmune diseases.

Huntington's Chorea

Autosomal dominant.
First presents in the thirties.
Choreiform movements, particularly of face.
Jerks and twitches may become violent.
Personality changes precede progressive dementia.
Invariably fatal; may take 10 to 20 years.

Hutchinson's Freckle
(Lentigo Maligna.)

On the face of the elderly.
Melanotic with marked junctional activity.
Involves deep layers of epidermis.
No dermal invasion.
Invasion and metastasis may occur after many years but relatively good prognosis.

Hutchinson's Tumour

Adrenal neuroblastoma.
Skull metastases.
Exophthalmos.
Periorbital discolouration.

Jacksonian Epilepsy

Focal epilepsy.
Involuntary twitching confined to one part of the body.
Spreads to involve adjacent areas.
Extent of spread varies.
May or may not lose consciousness.
May be left with transient paralysis of parts involved in attack (Todd's palsy).

Jefferson Fracture

Fracture of C1 (atlas) vertebra in four places.
Neurological complications unusual as nature of fracture effectively enlarges space available for the cord.

Johansson-Larsen's Disease

Partial avulsion of patellar ligament from lower pole of patella.
Traction tendonitis leads to ossification.

Kaposi's Sarcoma

Haemorrhagic sarcoma of skin.
Multiple lesions.
Each lesion multifocal.
May lead to lymphoedema and ulceration.
Occur also in gastrointestinal tract.
Malignant tumour of new blood vessels and large spindle cells.
Common in tropical Africa, in transplant patients on immunotherapy and as a complication of AIDS.

Kaposi's Varicelliform Eruption
(Eczema Herpeticum.)

Widespread skin lesion due to primary infection with herpes simplex virus in patient with pre-existing atopic dermatitis.

Katayama Fever

Acute schistosomiasis (Bilharzia).
Most frequent and severe with S. japonicum and S. mansoni.
3-8 weeks after infection in previously unexposed.
Resembles serum sickness.
Fever, chills, myalgia and urticarial rash.
Abdominal pain and splenomegaly.
Eosinophilia.
Headache, sweating and weakness.
Anorexia and diarrhoea.

Kienbock's Disease

Osteochondritis of the carpal lunate bone.
Predominantly male.
Does not have the age incidence typical of osteochondritis juvenilis.
Frequent history of trauma.
Pain and stiffness in wrist.

Kinnear-Wilson Disease
(v. Wilson Disease.)

Kissing Disease

Infectious mononucleosis (glandular fever).
Epstein-Barr virus transmitted in saliva.

Klumpke's Paralysis

Brachial plexus injury, usually at birth.
Mainly involving the lower trunk composed of C8 and T1.
Results in claw hand due to paralysis of intrinsic muscles.
Horner's syndrome may be associated due to sympathetic damage.

Kohler's Disease

Osteochondritis of the tarsal navicular bone.
Mainly males aged 3 to 8 years.
Pain in foot and limp.
Tender medial aspect of foot.
Radiologically navicular is dense, flattened to a disc.

Krabbe's Disease

Genetically determined enzyme disorder.
Results in lipid accumulation.
Signs appear at birth or early childhood.
Psychomotor retardation.
Peripheral neuropathy.
Retinal changes.
Skeletal deformities.

Krukenberg Tumour

Secondary ovarian malignant tumour.
Usually bilateral.
Primary usually stomach, colon or pancreas.
Doubts over transcoelomic spread as tumour surface smooth with no seedlings.
Sometimes no obvious gastrointestinal source.
Mucin secreting cells give characteristic "signet ring" appearance on microscopy.

Kugelberg-Welander Disease
(Spinal Muscular Atrophy.)

Neurogenic muscular atrophy.
Caused by abnormality of anterior horn cells.
Proximal muscles mainly involved, legs first.
Tendon reflexes absent.
If onset in infancy, severe and rapidly progressive.
The later the onset, the milder the course.

Kummell's Disease

Spondylitis following compression fracture of vertebra.

Kussmaul's Disease

Intermittent pain, swelling and infection in parotid and submandibular salivary glands.
Caused by mucinous plugs obstructing ducts.
Common in debilitated, irradiated and immunosuppressed patients.

Kyasanur Forest Fever

Arboviral infection (i.e. arthropod borne).
Transmitted by ticks.
Disease of India.
Fever with maculopapular rash.
Photophobia and pain in orbit.
Arthralgia and myalgia, often severe.
May develop encephalitis, haemorrhage and circulatory failure.

Ladd's Bands

Peritoneal bands associated with gastro-duodenal malrotation.
Cause duodenal obstruction.

Laennec's Cirrhosis
(Portal Cirrhosis.)

Micronodular cirrhotic changes of progressive fibrosis and nodular regeneration.
Characteristic of alcohol abuse.

Distortion of liver architecture producing portal-systemic vascular shunts.
Portal hypertension.
Haematemesis.
Liver failure.

Landouzy-Dejerine Dystrophy
(Facio-scapulo-humeral Muscular Dystrophy.)

Autosomal dominant muscle disorder.
Both sexes of any age; usually 12 to 14 year old.
Begins in facial muscles; difficulty in closing eyes, sucking, blowing.
Spreads to shoulder girdle.
Pelvic girdle may be affected years later.
Slow, irregular progression.
Compatible with long life.
Confirmed by electromyography or muscle biopsy.
Serum enzyme changes may precede clinical manifestations.

Landry's Paralysis

Acute ascending paralysis.
Variant of Guillain-Barre syndrome.
May also be presenting feature of acute poliomyelitis.

Lassa Fever

Caused by arenavirus, spread by rats (Mastomys natalensis), probably in their urine.
Human to human transmission also possible.
Limited to West Africa.

Fever and myalgia.
Bradycardia and hypotension.
Leucopenia.
Characteristic yellow pharyngeal exudate.
Hepato-renal failure.
Haemorrhage and circulatory failure.

Leber's Hereditary Optic Atrophy

Trait inherited via mitochondrial DNA.
Mostly young males - transmitted almost exclusively by female.
Neuropathy causing bilateral visual loss with central scotomata.
Usually acute onset.

Lederer's Anaemia
(Idiopathic Acquired Haemolytic Anaemia.)

May have alarmingly acute onset in children.
Fever, backache, abdominal pain, vomiting and diarrhoea.
Oliguria and haemoglobinuria.
Pallor and icterus.
Splenomegaly.
Spherocytosis with increased red cell fragility.
May mimic congenital spherocytosis but Coombs Test positive.
Complete recovery may follow blood transfusion.

Le Fort Fractures

Three classical fractures of mandible.

Legg-Calve-Perthes' Disease
(v. Perthes' Disease.)

Legionnaire's Disease
(Legionella Pneumonia.)

Legionella pneumophila transmitted via water droplets from infected cisterns in warm climates.
Gastrointestinal symptoms.
Mental confusion.
Spreading type of pneumonia.
Maybe cavitation and pleural effusion.
Hyponatraemia.
Proteinuria.
Occasionally fatal, especially in elderly and debilitated.

Leigh's Disease
(Subacute Necrotising Encephalopathy.)

Probably linked to thiamine deficiency.
Lethal disorder of infancy.
Psychomotor delay.
Myoclonus.
Ocular paralyses.
Respiratory disorders.

Lennert's Lymphoma

T-cell lymphoma.
Profusion of non-malignant epithelioid cells may give false appearance of granuloma.
May occur in the tonsils of the elderly.
Generalised lymphadenopathy and splenomegaly.

Leri's Disease
(Melorheostosis. Candle Bones.)

Pain and stiffness in one limb.
X-rays show linear patches of osteosclerosis.
Appear like congealed wax on side of burning candle.
May be associated with scleroderma.

Letterer-Siwe Disease

Eosinophilic granuloma.
May occur at any age but usually rapidly fatal disease of infancy.
Infant fails to thrive.
Fever.
Haemorrhagic seborrhoeic rash.
Lymphadenopathy.
Hepatosplenomegaly.
Bony lesions may be clinically silent.
Gland biopsy reveals eosinophil granuloma at malignant end of the scale.
Prognosis depends on extent of the disease.

Leydig Cell Tumour

Interstitial tumour of testis.
1.5% of all testicular tumours.
Raised gonadotrophin levels.
Gynaecomastia.
Impotence.
Change in hair distribution.
Atrophy of other testis.
Low malignancy and good prognosis.

Libman-Sach's Endocarditis

Verrucous endocarditis, seen on echocardiography.
Occurs in systemic lupus erythematosus.
Necrotic connective tissue erupts through endocardium.
Both sides of heart affected with mural and valvular vegetations.
Rarely severe enough to cause physical signs.

Littre's Hernia

Hernia, inguinal or femoral, containing a Meckel's diverticulum.

Lorain-Type Dwarfism

Hypopituitarism.
Deficiency of growth hormone.
Growth retardation leads to dwarfism.
Peculiar in that this type does not respond to growth hormone therapy.

Lou Gehrig's Disease
(Amyotrophic Lateral Sclerosis.)

Form of motor neurone disease.
Invariably fatal.
Upper motor neurone signs in legs.
Lower motor neurone signs in arms.
Wasting and weakness of small muscles of hand often first sign.
Fasciculation then wasting of limb muscles.
Onset 50 to 70 years.
May have rapid progression to death within 3 years.

Ludwig's Angina

Cellulitis floor of mouth and submandibular space.
Majority follow dental caries and root abscesses.
Streptococcus viridans and E. coli.
Respiratory obstruction.
Pus rarely found on incision.

Lyell's Disease
(Ritter's Disease. Scalded Skin Syndrome.)

Epidermal necrolysis due to toxins of staphylococcus type 71.
Acute skin infection develops into generalised skin exfoliation.
May also follow certain therapeutic drugs.
Slightest trauma results in loss of skin.

Lyme Disease

Infection with Spirochaete Borrelia Burgdorferi.
Bite of tick Ixodes.
Stage 1 - Flu like illness.
　　Pathognomonic erythema migrans.
Stage 2 - Involvement of skin, heart, joints and CNS.
　　Lasts days to months.
Stage 3 - Chronic or recurrent arthritis.

Lynch Type Tumours

Hereditary non-polyposis cancers of colon.
Autosomal dominant.
Chromosome 17 or 18 abnormality.
Clinically similar to sporadic cases though at younger age.

5% of all colorectal cancers.
Two types -
- Lynch Type 1 - susceptible to colonic cancers only.
- Lynch Type 2 - female family members susceptible also to breast and uterine cancers.

Madelung's Deformity

Lower radius curves forwards together with carpus and hand.
Ulna remains straight and projects on dorsum of wrist.
Usually due to post traumatic damage to growth cartilage.
May be congenital though not apparent until ten years old.

Majocchi's Granuloma

Inflamed papules lower leg.
Trichophyton infection of feet.
Commonly due to shaving legs.

Maladie de Reclus

Fibroadenosis of breast.
Multiple breast lumps.
May be associated with cysts.
Histologically proliferating ducts and acini in increased fibrous stroma.
Premenstrual pain.

Maladie de Roger

Symptomless child.
Normally developed.

Heart normal size.
Palpable systolic thrill left parasternal region.
Harsh systolic murmur fourth left interspace.
Caused by small congenital ventricular septal defect.
ECG normal.

Maltworker's Lung

Allergic pulmonary reaction to organic dust.
Aspergillus clavatus from malting barley.
Cellular exudates lead to small granulomatous lesions.
Impaired pulmonary compliance, ventilation and perfusion.
Prolonged exposure produces permanent damage.

Marburg Disease

Infection with Ebola virus.
May be transmitted human to human.
Fever, myalgia and headache.
Follicular rash starting on extensor aspects of limbs.
Lymphadenopathy.
Thrombocytopenia and bleeding.
Encephalitis.
Renal failure.
High mortality rate.

Marchiafava-Bignami Disease

Emotional disturbance.
Seizures.
Rigidity.
Paralysis.
Coma.

Death.
Closely associated with alcoholism.

Marion's Disease

Bladder neck obstruction.
Almost solely in boys.
Caused by fibro-elastosis in posterior urethra.
Rarely gives symptoms before one year.
Late diagnosis can lead to significant renal failure.

Marjolin's Ulcer

Squamous cell carcinoma developing in margin of chronic inflammatory ulcer.
Should be reserved for chronic leg ulcers.
Generally applied also to such conditions as old burns scars, osteomyelitis sinuses and tropical sores.

Maydl's Hernia

Hernia with three loops.
Two loops in hernial sac, intermediate loop back in abdominal cavity.
Loop in abdomen may strangulate without any external signs.

McArdle's Disease

Inherited autosomal recessive glycogen storage disorder.
Enzyme (phosphorylase) deficiency.
Aged 20 to 40 years.
Inability to perform strenuous exercise due to muscle cramp.
Best demonstrated by exercising forearm with inflated cuff on upper arm.

Myoglobinuria may occur.
Muscle weakness and wasting follow.

Meibomian Cyst
(Chalazion.)

Retention cyst of a tarsal gland on the eyelid.

Meleney's Burrowing Ulcer

Follows operation on intestinal or genital tract.
Subcutaneous infection with combined haemolytic microaerophilic streptococcus and staphylococcus.
Burrows deep into pelvis.
Very painful.

Meleney's Postoperative Synergistic Gangrene

Usually follows drainage of deep abscess.
Either peritoneal or pleural.
Spreading infection of skin.
Ill defined (cf. erysipelas).
Bright red margin.
Black central gangrenous slough.
Slough separates to leave granulating surface.

MEN 1.
(Multiple Endocrine Neoplasia. Wermer's Syndrome.)

Autosomal dominant.
Hyperparathyroidism.

Pancreatic tumours (gastrinoma; insulinoma).
Hyperinsulinism.
Anterior pituitary hyperplasia (acidophil or chromophobe adenomata).
Adrenal hyperplasia and carcinoid tumours (rare).
Thyroid tumours (rare).
Zollinger-Ellison and Verner-Morrison syndromes may coexist.

MEN 2
(Multiple Endocrine Neoplasia. Sipple's Syndrome.)

Thyroid medullary carcinoma.
Phaeochromocytoma.
Multiple neuromata.
Hyperparathyroidism.
Marfan-like characteristics.
Cushing's syndrome (rare).

Menetrier's Disease

Protein losing gastropathy.
Extreme hypertrophic gastric folds, largely sparing the antrum.
Gastric hypersecretion.
Low acid content.
Chronic gastro-intestinal plasma protein loss.
Severe hypoproteinaemia results.
May be premalignant.

Meniere's Disease

Recurrent attacks of vertigo.
40 to 60 years.

Unknown aetiology.
Immediate cause is excessive endolymph in membranous labyrinth (inner ear).
Sudden onset with sweating, weakness and fainting.
Preceding feeling of fullness in ear.
May be profound with vomiting.
Last few minutes to several hours.
Episodic but generally progressive.
Progressive sensorineural deafness, 25% bilateral.
Tinnitus.
Rotary nystagmus and ataxia.
Often associated with migraine.

Mikulicz's Disease

Enlargement of salivary and lachrymal glands.
No systemic disorder.
Regarded as variant of Sjogren's disease.

Milroy's Disease

Primary lymphoedema.
May be familial, M : F :: 1 : 2.
Predominantly lower limb.
Onset congenital to early adult life (lymphoedema praecox).
May appear in middle aged (lymphoedema tarda).
No radiologically demonstrable lymphatic obstruction.
Possibly due to lymphatic aplasia.
May co-exist with Pierre-Robin syndrome.

Minkowski-Chauffard Disease

Hereditory microspherocytosis.
Red cell fragility.
Haemolytic jaundice.

Mollaret's Meningitis

Recurrent lymphocytic meningitis.
Fever.
No detectable cause.

Monckeberg's Sclerosis
(Medial Sclerosis.)

Old age.
Occasionally in healthy young adults.
Degeneration in muscular coat of medium sized arteries.
Calcification in hyalinised tunica media to give "pipe stem" arteries.
Lumen not unduly narrowed.
May occur in rings.
Normal intima.
Little clinical significance.
Pressure required to occlude artery may be greater than systolic blood pressure.

Mondor's Disease
(String Phlebitis.)

Skin tethering on chest wall.
Sclerosing angiitis or phlebitis.

May extend on to female breast.
Mimics tethering of scirrhous carcinoma of breast.

Monteggia Fracture

Fracture of ulnar shaft with dislocation of head of radius.
Dislocation may be forwards or backwards, depending on angulation of fracture.

Morgagni Hernia

Through defect in diaphragm due to failure of fusion between central and lateral muscular elements anteriorly.
Retrosternal hernia into chest.
Rarely cause respiratory problems.
Occasional intestinal obstruction.

Morton's Metatarsalgia
(Digital Neuroma.)

Enlarged, inflamed digital nerve between two metatarsal heads.
Usually third and fourth metatarsals.
Middle aged patients, women 40 to 50 years.
Pain localised to one interdigital cleft, usually third.
Acute pain on lateral compression of foot.

Mounier-Kuhn Disease
(Tracheobronchomegaly.)

Congenital abnormality.
May present as respiratory distress in infancy.
Usually becomes apparent in adult life.

Circumference of trachea and bronchi increased.
Problems arise from cartilagenous deformities.

Mule Spinner's Cancer

Epithelioma of abdominal wall and scrotum.
Lancashire cotton mills.
Chemical carcinogens in shale oil seeping through clothing.

Murray Valley Fever

Arboviral infection (i.e. arthropod borne).
Transmitted by mosquito.
Fever with maculopapular rash.
Photophobia and pain in orbit.
Arthralgia and myalgia, often severe.
May develop encephalitis, haemorrhage and circulatory failure.

Niemann-Pick Disease

Inherited enzyme (shingomyelinase) disorder.
Results in phospholipid accumulation.
Hepatosplenomegaly.
Mental retardation.
Yellow skin.
May have cherry red macular spot.
Characteristic "foamy" cells on histology.
Five variants.
Acute infantile most common.
Usually die before aged 4 years.
Chronic visceral type has no mental or neurological problems.

Norrie's Disease

Sex linked hereditary blindness.
Bilateral non malignant retinal tumours.
Deafness.
Mentally retarded.

Ollier's Disease
(Dyschondroplasia.)

May run in families.
Small rests of epiphyseal cells remain in metaphyseal end of long bone.
As epiphysis grows, ends of long bones become enlarged.
Longitudinal growth is impaired with marked shortening.
Asymmetrical extremities.
Produces enchondromata in hands and feet.
Deformities may range from minimal to grotesque.

Omsk Haemorrhagic Fever

Arboviral infection (i.e. arthropod borne).
Transmitted by ticks.
Fever with maculopapular rash.
Photophobia and pain in orbit.
Arthralgia and myalgia, often severe.
May develop encephalitis, haemorrhage and circulatory failure.

Ondine's Curse

Congenital central hypoventilation syndrome.
Neural crest abnormality results in aganglionosis.
Impaired autonomic control of respiration.
Requires diaphragmatic pacing.

Oroya Fever
(v. Carrion's Disease.)

Osgood-Schlatter's Disease
(Schlatter's Disease.)

Osteochondritis of tibial tubercle.
Commonest site for osteochondritis.
Usually boys aged 12 to 16 years.
Perhaps related to repeated trauma giving a traction apophysitis or stress fracture.
Fragmentation with separation from tibia.
Resolves spontaneously with rest from violent sport.

Osler's Disease

Hereditary haemorrhagic telangiectasia.
Autosomal dominant disorder.
Congenital defect in capillaries.
Epistaxis.
Gastro-intestinal bleeding.
Occasional pulmonary arterio-venous anomalies.

Osler-Vaquez Disease
(Polycythaemia Rubra Vera.)

Commonest in males over 40 years.
May be symptomless.
Lassitude, headaches, epistaxis.
High colour with suffused facies.
Splenomegaly.
May present as peripheral vascular disease.
Average survival 10 years.

Paget's Disease of Bone
(Osteitis deformans.)

Middle aged or elderly of either sex, more commonly men.
Widespread, paatchy bone disorder.
Most commonly involving pelvis, femur, tibia, lumbar spine and skull.
Decalcification and softening followed by recalcification and hardening.
Processes may coexist in different sites.
Usually starts in one bone.
Rarely affects whole skeleton.
Bony thickening and deformities which may be gross.
Skull thickening may cause deafness.
Normal serum calcium and greatly raised alkaline phosphatase.
Spontaneous fractures.
Deformities lead to secondary osteoarthroses.
Raised bone temperature in vascular, resorptive stage.
Vascularity may be so gross as to produce effects similar to an arterio-venous fistula.
Occasionally, severe cases develop bone sarcoma.

Paget's Disease of Nipple

Eczematous lesion of nipple and areolar.
Usually in the elderly.
Exudes clear or bloodstained fluid.
Large round hydropic cells on microscopy of deeper epidermal layers.
Widely held now as example of carcinoma-in-situ.
May precede but usually signifies the presence of underlying schirrous carcinoma of breast.

Similar lesions may occur on vulva, anus, penis and axilla when not always associated with frank carcinoma.

Paget's Recurring Fibroma
(Desmoid Tumour.)

Most commonly in rectus sheath of parous women.
No capsule.
Invades surrounding muscle.
Well differentiated histologically.
Does not metastasise.
Recurs if not adequately removed.

Pancoast Tumour
(Pancoast Syndrome)

Apical bronchial carcinoma.
May show rib lysis.
Pain in arm due to direct invasion of C8 and T1 nerve roots.
Often associated with Horner's syndrome.

Panner's Disease

Osteochondritis dissecans of the elbow.
Under age of 12 years.
Ossification centre of the capitulum is fragmented.

Parkinson's Disease
(Paralysis Agitans.)

Tremor of extremities, worse in arm than leg.
Subdued at first by purposeful movement.

Onset usually 50 to 70 years.
Muscle rigidity develops to make purposeful movement difficult (dyskinesia).
Rigidity may include jerky "cog wheel" movement.
Rhythmical movement of thumb towards fingers (pill rolling).
Short shuffling steps.
Uncontrolled acceleration (festination).
Difficult to stand erect, speak, write or focus eyes.
Basal ganglia deficient in the neurotransmitter dopamine.
May be a sequel to encephalitis lethargica.
Onset after encephalitis may be sudden and progress rapid.
One third of cases have intellectual deterioration (subcortical dementia).

Parry's Disease
(v. Grave's Disease.)

Pel-Ebstein Fever

Intermittent fever in Hodgkin's lymphoma.
Pyrexia 39° C and above for several days.
Normal temperature between bouts.

Perthes' Disease
(Osteochondritis Juvenilis. Coxa Plana.
Legg-Calve-Perthes' Disease.)

Aged 2 to 10 years.
M : F :: 5 : 1.
10% bilateral.
Not infective.
Considered avascular necrosis of femoral head due to thrombosis of minute veins.

Limp, painless or painful; pain may be referred to knee.
Limited abduction and internal rotation of hip.
Femoral head first small, dark and irregular on X-ray.
Fragmentation follows with dense areas surrounded by osteoporosis.
Coxa plana; femoral head becomes flattened and deformed.
Predisposes to osteoarthritis.

Peyronie's Disease

Fibrotic changes in corpus cavernosa of penis.
Pain and distortion.
Aetiology unknown.
10% have Dupuytren's contracture.

Pick's Disease

M : F :: 1 : 2.
Strong genetic tendency.
Early personality changes with euphoria.
Usually starts in the fifties but may also in twenties.
Fatuous and apathetic.
Loss of insight.
Incontinence.
Later amnesia.
Intellectual deterioration.
Patchy atrophy of frontal and temporal cerebral lobes.
Leads to gross dementia and death.

Pick's Disease
(Chronic Constrictive Pericarditis.)

Majority of cases in children tuberculous in origin.
Adults often idiopathic.
May follow traumatic haemopericadium.
Raised venous pressure.
Impaired cardiac filling.
Diminished stroke volume.
Gross ascites and hepatomegaly.
Feeble heart sounds.

Pink Disease
(Infantile Acrodynia.)

Probably due to ingestion of mercury.
Much less common now since use of calomel discontinued.
May occur in children never exposed to mercury.
Onset usually during "teething" period.
Irritable and sleepless.
Severe anorexia.
Excessive sweating.
Hypotonia.
Marked photophobia (head buried in the pillows).
Extremities grossly hyperaemic but cold.
Palms and soles desquamate.
Hypertension.
Susceptible to chest infections, sometimes fatal.

Plummer's Disease
(Toxic Multinodular Goitre.)

Hyperthyroidism in nodular goitre (cf. Graves disease).

Usually over 50 years old.
Goitre usually present years before onset of toxic symptoms.
Exophthalmos rare.
May also have obstructive symptoms.

Pompe Disease

Autosomal recessive metabolic disorder.
Glycogen storage disease due to lysosomal enzyme deficiency.
Infantile form of myopathy.
Onset in early weeks.
Anorexia, dyspnoea and failure to thrive.
Gross hypotonia.
Extreme cardiomegaly.
Presents with cardiac failure and hepatomegaly.
Death inevitable before 18 months.

Pott's Disease

Tuberculous disease of spine.
Starts in metaphysis.
Rapidly involves epiphysis and neighbouring joints.
Extensive local destruction including intervertebral discs.
Vertebral collapse.
Angulation of spine (gibbus).

Pott's Fracture

External rotation fracture dislocation of ankle joint.
Oblique fracture of fibula.
Avulsion fracture of medial malleolus or rupture of deltoid ligament.

Joint invariably involved.
May occur with or without diastasis of inferior tibio-fibular joint.

Pott's Puffy Tumour

Oedema of scalp.
Due to underlying osteomyelitis of skull with extradural pus.
Usually from frontal sinusitis, middle ear disease or compound fracture.

Pringle's Disease.
(v. Bourneville's Disease.)

Prinzmetal's Angina
(Variant Angina.)

Typical anginal symptoms.
Occur capriciously.
Caused by coronary artery spasm.
Accompanied by transient ST elevation on ECG.

Pyle's Disease
(Metaphysial Dysplasia.)

Autosomal recessive.
Genu valgum due to failure of bone modelling.
X-rays show typical "bottle shape" to distal femur and proximal tibia.

Q Fever

Caused by Rickettsia like organism, Coxiella burnetii.

Carried by many insects, ticks and animals.
Commoner in rural communities.
Pyrexia with myalgia, headaches and sweating.
Myocarditis.
Hepatitis.
Osteomyelitis.
Endocarditis with sterile blood culture.
Weil-Felix reaction negative.
Some minor cases resolve spontaneously.
More severe cases die from encephalitis or endocarditis.

Queensland Tick Typhus

Infection with Rickettsia australis.
Tick borne.
Lymphadenopathy in region of bite.
Maculopapular rash, first on wrists and ankles, then generalised.
Hepato-splenomegaly.
Cutaneous and subcutaneous haemorrhages.

Randall's Plaques
(Nephrocalcinosis.)

Dystrophic calcification in renal papillae.
Ulcerate through pelvic epithelium.
Form nidus for formation of renal calculi.

Raynaud's Disease

Raynaud's phenomenon with no evidence of vascular or other organic disease.
Usually young females.
50% family history.

Symmetrical, bilateral finger blanching due to digital vascular spasm.
Exaggerated response to cold.
Transient cyanosis on rewarming followed by red, painful reactive hyperaemia.

Raynaud's Phenomenon

Identical features with Raynaud's disease but indicative of some other disorder.
Scleroderma.
Thromboangeitis obliterans.
Obstruction to axillary or brachial artery.
Polyarteritis.
Systemic lupus erythematosus.
Sjogren's disease.
Occupational use of vibrating tools.

Reidel's Struma
(Ligneous Thyroiditis.)

Rare thyroid disorder.
Mainly men.
Painless, stony hard thyroid enlargement.
Adherent to surrounding structures.
Pressure effects may be severe.
Histology shows infiltration with dense fibrous tissue.
Retroperitoneal fibrosis may also occur.

Reinke's Oedema

Fluid collection in loose epithelial space of vocal cords (Reinke's space).

Exact cause unknown.
May follow respiratory or sinus infection.
May be mechanical from over use or misuse of vocal cords.
More frequently in women or children (cf. chronic laryngitis in males).

Reiter's Disease

Non specific urethritis.
Conjunctivitis.
Seronegative arthritis in weight bearing joints.
Follows 1 to 3 weeks after sexual exposure or attack of bacterial dysentery.
M : F :: 50 : 1.
Male predominance may be partially explained by urethritis going undiagnosed in women.
May also have fever, weight loss and vaso motor changes in feet.
Arthritis may persist after conjunctivitis and urethritis have subsided.
Untreated uveitis may lead to glaucoma.
Often associated with chlamydial infection.
Thickened plantar skin.

Remak Paralysis

Wrist drop and other motor neuropathies.
Lead poisoning.

Rich's Focus

Cerebral subcortical tuberculous focus.
Part of miliary spread.

May rupture into subarachnoid space to give tuberculous meningitis.

Richter's Hernia

Hernia involving only part of the bowel's circumference.
Easy to overlook in absence of intestinal obstruction.

Rift Valley Fever

Arbovirus transmitted from sheep and goats by mosquito (culex pipieus).
East and South Africa.
Fever.
Retinal changes.
Jaundice.
Haemorrhages.
Meningo-encephalitis, often fatal.

Ritter's Disease
(v. Lyell's Disease.)

Rocky Mountain Spotted Fever

Tick borne typhus, caused by Rickettsia rickettsi.
Parts of USA and South America.
Lymphadenopathy in region of bite.
Maculopapular rash, first on wrists and ankles, then generalised.
Hepato-splenomegaly.
Cutaneous and subcutaneous haemorrhages.
Gangrene of fingers, toes and genitalia.
Weil-Felix reaction negative to OXK.

Rosai-Dorfmann Disease

Unknown aetiology.
Massive, bilateral, painless, cervical lymphadenopathy.
Fever.
Weight loss.
Histology shows sinus histiocytosis.
One third have extranodal involvement of orbit, upper respiratory tract, skin and bones.
Spontaneous resolution after protracted course.

Ross River Fever

Arbovirus transmitted by mosquito.
Australia.
Fever with maculopapular rash.
Photophobia and pain in orbit.
Arthralgia and myalgia, often severe.
May develop encephalitis, haemorrhage and circulatory failure.

Schatzki's Ring

Mucosal ridge at gastro-oesophageal junction.
Mostly asymptomatic.
Associated with hiatus hernia.
Not associated with oesophagitis.
Thought to be responsible for acute obstruction by food bolus (steak house syndrome).

Scheuermann's Disease
(Adolescent Kyphosis.)

Osteochondritis of vertebral body epiphyses.
Usually multiple in thoracic region.
Puberty.
Backache.
Round shouldered.
Leads to wedging later in life.

Schilder's Disease
(Encephalitis Periaxialis Diffusa.)

Extensive cerebral demyelination - cause unknown.
Children.
Intellectual and visual impairment.
Progressive spastic weakness all four limbs.
Sensory loss.
Blindness.
Incontinence.
Aphasia.
Epilepsy.
Pseudobulbar palsy.
Pathologically multifocal lesions akin to those in multiple sclerosis.
Death within a year or so.

Schimmelbusch's Disease

Fibroadenosis of breast.
Multiple breast lumps.
May be associated with cysts.

Histologically proliferating ducts and acini in increased fibrous stroma.
Premenstrual pain.

Schlatter's Disease
(v. Osgood-Schlatter's Disease.)

Semiliki Forest Fever

Arboviral infection (i.e. arthropod borne) transmitted by mosquito.
Africa.
Fever with maculopapular rash.
Photophobia and pain in orbit.
Arthralgia and myalgia, often severe.
May develop encephalitis, haemorrhage and circulatory failure.

Sever's Disease

Osteochondritis of the calcaneal epiphysis.
May follow trauma via the Achilles tendon.
Mainly males aged 10 to 13 years old.
Common cause of painful heels in children.

Silo-Filler's Disease

Obliterative bronchiolitis.
Follows inhalation of industrial nitrous peroxide.

Simmond's Disease
(Pituitary Cachexia.)

Complete destruction of pituitary (adenohypophysis).

Extreme wasting.
Apathy.
Fatal without treatment.

Sindbis Fever

Arboviral infection (i.e. arthropod borne) transmitted by mosquito.
Africa.
Fever with maculopapular rash.
Photophobia and pain in orbit.
Arthralgia and myalgia, often severe.
May develop encephalitis, haemorrhage and circulatory failure.

Singer's Nodes

Nodules on vocal cords.
Most commonly in children.
Result from excessive vocal use.
Fibrous tissue covered with epithelium.

Smith's Fracture
(Reversed Colles Fracture.)

Result of forced flexion injury to the wrist.
Usually young adult.

Spiegler-Fendt Sarcoid
(Pseudolymphoma of Skin.)

Cutaneous nodules of lymphoid tissue.
Histologically resembles closely nodular lymphocytic lymphoma.
Never develops into overt malignancy.

Similar to pseudolymphoma that occurs in the orbit.

Spielmeyer-Vogt Disease
(v. Batten's Disease)

Spigelian Hernia

Hernia through the semilunar line, lateral to the rectus abdominis.
Spreads deep to the external oblique muscle.
Occasionally lies within rectus sheath.

Spitz Naevus
(Benign Juvenile Melanoma.)

Typically appear suddenly in children or adolescents as pink or red papules or nodules.
May be deeply pigmented in dark complexioned.
Made up of spindle and epithelioid cells but mitoses and atypical appearances may be mistaken for malignant melanoma.
Differentiation histologically may be difficult.

Sprengel Deformity

Congenitally high scapula.

St. Anthony's Fire

Severe post herpetic neuralgia.
Follows attack of shingles.
More severe in the elderly.

Steinert's Disease
(Dystrophia Myotonica.)

Autosomal dominant.
20 to 30 year old.
Cataracts.
Baldness.
Ptosis and facial weakness.
Gynaecomastia.
Cardiac abnormalities.
Depressed or absent tendon reflexes.
Testicular atrophy.

Stewart Nasal Granuloma

Probably autoimmune.
Malignant granuloma.
Limited to the skull.
Similar to that which causes ulceration of the nose and adjacent structures.
Characterised by pleomorphic histiocyte infiltration.

Still's Disease
(Juvenile Chronic Arthritis.)

Typical polyarticular juvenile arthritis but commencing with generalised systemic upset.
Lymphadenopathy.
Hepatosplenomegaly.
Pleurisy, pericarditis and iridocyclitis.
Fever with myalgia and arthralgia.
Variable symmetrical polyarthritis.

Most commonly between 1 and 5 years.
Rheumatoid factor negative.
25% go on to have severe chronic polyarthritis.

St. Louis Fever

Arboviral infection (i.e. arthropod borne) transmitted by mosquito.
Fever with maculopapular rash.
Photophobia and pain in orbit.
Arthralgia and myalgia, often severe.
May develop encephalitis, haemorrhage and circulatory failure.

St. Vitus Dance
(v. Sydenham's Chorea.)

Sudek's Atrophy
(Traumatic Osteoporosis.)

Painful bony decalcification in region of trauma.
Cause unknown.
Wrist and hand in Colles fracture.
Ankle and foot in Pott's fracture.
May follow minor injury.
Patient protects painful limb.
Disuse aggravates condition.
Accompanied by vasomotor changes.
Skin first red and warm, later cold and shiny.

Sutton's Naevus
(Halo Naevus.)

Spontaneous regression of a naevus.
May leave surrounding area of depigmentation.
Histology shows lymphatic infiltration.
Not a sign of malignancy.

Sydenham's Chorea
(St. Vitus Dance.)

Commonest in adolescent girls.
May follow streptococcal throat infection.
Associated with rheumatic fever.
Choreiform movements particularly extremities and face.
Emotionally unstable.
Most recover within one month though recurrence is frequent.
Pregnancy may trigger recurrence.
May predispose to valvular heart disease.

Symes Amputation

Amputation of foot and ankle joint.
Bone end covered with heel flap of tough skin and subcutaneous tissue.
End bearing stump.

Takayasu's Disease
(Pulseless Disease. Aortic Arch Syndrome.)

Arteritis of aortic arch, probably of autoimmune origin.
Progressive obstruction to major branches.
Common in young Oriental (Japanese) women.

Pulses absent in arms, head and neck.
May rarely involve descending aorta and pulmonary artery.
Muscular weakness.
Cerebral ischaemia.
Headaches and syncope.
Visual disturbances leading to blindness.
Poor prognosis.
70% present with fever, malaise, myalgia and arthralgia.

Tangier Disease
(Familial Alpha-lipoprotein Deficiency.)

Lipoprotein deficiency results in low plasma cholesterol levels.
Gross enlargement of tonsils which are orange in colour.
Disabling peripheral neuropathy develops later.

Tay-Sachs Disease
(Amaurotic Familial Idiocy.)

Autosomal recessive enzyme disorder (hexosaminidase A).
Results in abnormal accumulation of ganglioside in cerebral grey matter.
Only in Ashkenazi Jews.
Both sexes.
Death inevitable in early childhood.
Infantile - within 6 months.
Late infantile - onset 2 to 3 years.
Previously normal child becomes limp and unresponsive.
Exaggerated startle response due to hyperacusis is early sign.
Seizures.
Hypotonia.
Visual problems lead to blindness within one year.
Characteristic cherry red spot in macula.

Rapid increase in cranial size due to cerebral enlargement (not hydrocephalus).

Thomsen's Disease
(Myotonia Congenita.)

Autosomal dominant.
Unknown aetiology.
Appears early childhood.
Slow muscle relaxation after contraction.
No muscle weakness.
Legs most severely affected.
Difficulty in relaxing grip and opening eyes.
Prolonged muscle contraction after percussion.
Not life threatening.

Todd's Palsy

Transient paralysis of part recovering from attack of Jacksonian epilepsy.
May last for minutes, perhaps hours.

Trevor's Disease
(Dysplasia Epiphysealis Hemimelica.)

Dysplasia affecting only one limb and only one half of each epiphysis.
Usually ankle or knee.
Child, usually male.
Bony swelling on one side of joint only.

Vincent's Angina
(Ulcerative Stomatitis.)

Malnourished adults with bad dental hygiene.
Ulceration of gums, palate, lips and inner cheek.
Grey slough with surrounding erythema.
Spirochaetes and fusiform bacilli.
Infectious.

Virchow Triad

The three factors involved in thrombosis.
1. The vessel wall, especially the endothelium.
2. The blood flow.
3. The blood constituents, especially platelets and clotting factors.

Volkmann's Contracture

Fibrous replacement of muscle in region of a fracture.
Usually secondary to ischaemia.
Fibrous replacement more intense if venous occlusion also.
Commonest in muscles of forearm after supracondylar fracture of humerus.
Inability to extend fingers with wrist dorsiflexed.
May have distal impaired sensation.

von Gierke's disease

Hereditary autosomal recessive trait.
Children with glycogen storage disease.
Enzyme deficiency of glucose-6-phosphatase.
Detectable in liver, kidney and intestine.
Gross hepatomegaly.

Hypoglycaemic fits.
Stunted growth and osteoporosis.
Gouty tophi and xanthomata.
High mortality in early years.
Severe gout in those who survive into adulthood.
Adult survivors prone to malignant hepatoma.

von Hippel-Lindau Disease

Genetic abnormality on short arm of chromosome 3.
Autosomal dominant disorder of embryonic ectoderm.
70% develop renal cell carcinoma by 60 years.
Tendency to bilateral and multicentric disease.
Renal cell carcinoma is part of a complex of diseases including -
    multiple haemangioblastomata, commonly cerebellar or spinal,
    retinal angioma,
    renal cysts,
    pancreatic cysts,
    phaeochromocytoma.

von Recklinghausen's Disease
(Neurofibromatosis.)

Autosomal dominant and slowly progressive.
Fibromata of neurilemmal sheath.
Peripheral nerves, nerve roots and cranial nerves.
May be associated with glioma, meningioma and phaeochromocytoma.
Cafe-au-lait skin spots, particularly in axillae.
Cutaneous fibromata.
Benign, rounded, discrete tumours.
Occasional plexiform neuroma.

Eighth cranial nerve tumour.
Bone involvement may give kyphoscoliosis.

von Recklinghausen's Disease of Bone
(Osteitis Fibrosa Cystica.)

Severe case of hyperparathyroidism.
Now a rarity.
Osteoclastomata give X-Ray appearances of bone cysts.
Responds to Vitamin D therapy only after parathroidectomy.

von Willebrand's Disease
(Pseudohaemophilia B.)

Congenital autosomal dominant blood disorder.
Deficiency of factor 8 which facilitates platelet adherence to collagen.
Either sex.
Prolonged bleeding time.
Abnormal bruising.
Prolonged bleeding.
Post partum haemorrhage due to abrupt fall in factor 8 level on termination of pregnancy.
Acquired type may occur rarely after multiple blood transfusions or in autoimmune disorders.

Waldenstrom's Macroglobulinaemia

Commoner in elderly males.
Paraproteinaemia with high serum globulin.
Marrow infiltrated with neoplastic lymphocytes.
Bleeding from mucous membranes.

Anaemia.
May develop a hyperviscosity syndrome with visual and neurological symptoms.
Slow progress to autoimmune deficiency and susceptibility to infections.
Many are asymptomatic for years.
Majority survive 2 to 5 years, some living considerably longer.

Warthin's Tumour
(Papillary Cystadenoma Lymphomatosa.)

An adenolymphoma, almost exclusive to the parotid gland.
Smooth swelling in tail of gland.
Benign.
Malignant change rare.
Slow growing, often asymptomatic.
May feel cystic.
Often bilateral.

Wegener's Disease

Adults of either sex.
Necrotising vasculitis, both arteries and veins, particularly pulmonary.
Granulomatous lesions of upper respiratory tract.
Focal or diffuse glomerulonephritis.
Mot respond to treatment.
Death usually from respiratory infection or renal failure.

Weil's Disease

Leptospira icterohaemorrhagiae transmitted in rats' urine.

Spirochaetes can penetrate skin abrasions or mucosa.
Immersion in canals or stagnant water.
Fever and headache.
Severe myalgia.
Transient meningism.
Hepatitis with jaundice.
May progress to acute liver failure.
Renal tubular necrosis and renal failure.
Myocarditis with arrhythmias and cardiac failure.
Mortality 15 - 20%.

Werding-Hoffman Disease
(Spinal Muscular Atrophy.)

Hereditary motor neuropathy.
Muscular atrophy and weakness.
Caused by abnormality of anterior horn cells.
Shoulder and pelvic girdles most affected.
Onset in infancy.
"Floppy" baby with respiratory problems.
Severe and rapidly progressive, particularly in first year of life.
Death from respiratory failure before 18 months of age.

Wernicke's Aphasia
(Amnestic Aphasia.)

Speech defect.
Affects fluency, comprehension, repetition and writing.
Caused by lesion in left anterior temporal lobe.

Wernicke's Encephalopathy

Encephalopathy due to thiamine deficiency.
Europe and North America.
May present acutely when rapidly fatal if untreated.
Usually alcoholic.
More rarely malnutrition (e.g. prisoners of war).
Quietly confused with gross memory defect for recent events.
Bilateral symmetrical ophthalmoplegia.
Nystagmus.
Ataxia.
Polyneuropathy.

West Nile Fever

Arboviral infection (i.e. arthropod borne) transmitted by mosquito.
Fever with maculopapular rash.
Photophobia and pain in orbit.
Arthralgia and myalgia, often severe.
May develop encephalitis, haemorrhage and circulatory failure.

Whipple's Disease

Middle aged men.
One of group of inflammatory joint diseases with negative IgM factor.
Migratory oligo-articular though may be polyarticular and symmetrical.
Sacroiliitis and ankylosing spondylitis may occur.
Skin pigmentation.
Also have abdominal pain, steatorrhoea and weight loss.
Protein losing gastroenteropathy.
Oedema with low plasma proteins.
Small bowel biopsy diagnostic.

Wilkie's Disease

Compression of fourth part of duodenum between superior mesenteric vessels and spine.
Predisposing factors are acute weight loss and plaster jacket immobilisation.

Wilm's Tumour
(Nephroblastoma.)

Originates in embryonic kidney.
Contains both epithelial and connective tissues.
Pluripotential; may contain bone, cartilage, fat and striated muscle.
Various stages of differentiation.
Second most common malignant renal tumour.
Left more common than right; 10% bilateral.
Before aged 10 years.
Often presents in first year.
Abdominal mass.
Haematuria only in late stages.
Metastasises via lymph and blood.
Radiosensitive and responsive to chemotherapy.

Wilson's Disease
(Kinnier Wilson's Disease. Hepato-Lenticular Degeneration.)

Autosomal recessive copper metabolism disorder.
Abnormality of both absorption and excretion.
Normal at birth.
Steady increase in copper level in liver, basal ganglia and eyes.
Onset of symptoms 5 - 30 years.

Hepatic disease in children.
Basal ganglia symptoms in adolescence -
 choreoathetosis
 Parkinsonism
 progressive dementia.
Kayser-Fleischer rings (copper) in cornea require slit lamp examination.
Haemolysis.
Renal tubular damage.
Prognosis good if treated before irreparable damage.

Wool Sorters Disease

Infection with anthrax by inhalation of Bacillus anthracis.
Onset with acute laryngitis.
Virulent haemorrhagic bronchopneumonia follows.

Syndromes

Achard-Thiers Syndrome

Diabetes mellitus.
Hirsutism.
Occur concurrently in postmenopausal women.
Suggested higher incidence of uterine cancer.

Acquired Immune Deficiency Syndrome
(AIDS)

Impairment of immune system by infection with retro virus (HIV).
Bloodstream infection from certain tissue fluids from carrier.
Long incubation period - average 8 years.
Two strains of HIV.
HIV1 - U.S.A., Europe and most of Africa.
HIV2 - West Africa.
Mainly male homosexuals, intravenous drug addicts, recipients of infected blood transfusion.
May spread by heterosexual intercourse and to the foetus.
Early symptoms include intermittent fever, fatigue, diarrhoea, weight loss, malaise and lymphadenopathy.
Later prone to any form of infection.
Prone to tumour formation, particularly Kaposi's sarcoma.

Adair-Dighton Syndrome
(Osteogenesis Imperfecta.)

Autosomal dominant.
Fragile bones.
Blue sclera and teeth.
Short legs.
Cleft palate.

Adam's Syndrome

Dementia with ataxia and incontinence.
Enlarged cerebral ventricles.
No cerebral atrophy.
CSF blockage due to trauma, meningitis or subarachnoid heamorrhage.

Adrenogenital Syndrome

Endocrine disorder.
Excessive production of androgens by adrenal cortex.
Effects accentuated by increased ACTH production by pituitary.
Melanin skin pigmentation.
Hypertension.
Associated hormonal disturbances.
In infant males - virilism with body hair, deep voice, small testes, large penis.
In infant females - Masculine like genitals (pseudohermaphrodites).
In adult male - may go unnoticed.
In adult female - virilism with facial and body hair, atrophic breasts, acne, enlarged clitoris, deep voice, amenorrhoea and male musculature.

Adson's Syndrome
(v. Cervical Rib Syndrome.)

Ahumada-del Castillo Syndrome

Amenorrhoea and galactorrhoea in women who have never been pregnant.
50% frequency of detectable pituitary tumours.

Aicardi's Syndrome

X chromosome disorder.
Females only.
Lethal in utero for males.
Convulsions during which infant's head bends forwards as if bowing (salaam attacks).
Retinal abnormalities.
Visual impairment.
Mentally and physically retarded.
Vertebral abnormalities.
Scoliosis.
Hand deformities.
Rarely live to teenage.

Albright's Syndrome
(v. Albright's Hereditary Osteodystrophy.)

Alpers Syndrome
(Christensen-Krabbe Disease.)

Familial.
Progressive degeneration cerebral cortex.
White matter is spared.
Onset infancy or before five years.
Microcephaly.
Myoclonus.
Dementia.
Death.

Alport Syndrome

Boys more severely affected than girls.
Family history of nephritis.
Sensorineural deafness.
Severe, progressive form in males; death from uraemia before age of 40.
Females rarely die from renal failure.

Alstrom Syndrome

Lawrence-Moon-Biedl syndrome without mental retardation and polydactyly.

Angelman's Syndrome
(Happy Puppets.)

Chromosome 15 disorder.
Appears in early childhood.
Jerky and incoordinated arm and leg movements.
Hand flapping.
Associated with bursts of laughter.
Speech difficulties.
Fits - tending to improve.
Large mouth with protruding tongue.

Aortic Arch Syndrome
(Takayasu's Disease. Pulseless Disease.)

Arteritis of aortic arch, probably of autoimmune origin.
Progressive obstruction to major branches.
Common in young Oriental women (Takayasu's disease).
Impaired blood supply to head, neck and upper trunk.

Cerebral ischaemia.
Syncope.
Headaches.
Blindness.
Muscular weakness.
Poor prognosis.

Apert's Syndrome
(Acrocephalosyndactyly.)

Rare hereditary disorder.
Premature closure of cranial coronal suture.
Results in wide, high, short front to back skull (acrocephaly).
Bulging eyes due to shallow orbits.
Narrow palate, sometimes cleft.
Bony fusion of digits.
One third show mental retardation.

Arnold-Chiari Syndrome

Herniation of part of cerebellum through foramen magnum.
Results in dilatation of spinal cord's central canal.
Dissociated sensory loss.
Loss of pain and temperature sensation.
Other modalities preserved.
Trophic lesions from burns and trauma to hands.
Painless, disorganised (Charcot) joints.
Upper motor neurone signs in legs.

Ascher's Syndrome

Goitre.

Hypertrophy of upper eye lid (blepharochalasia).
Hypertrophy of upper lip.

Asperger's Syndrome

M : F :: 7 : 1
Children with some autistic features.
Difficulty in social adjustments.
Self absorbed.
Happier with rigidly applied routines.
Speech difficulties.
Clumsy.
Inappropriate facial expressions.
Language skills and intelligence more or less normal.

Avellis Syndrome

Unilateral paralysis of palate, pharynx and vocal cords.
Brainstem infarction involving vagal nucleus.

Banti's Syndrome

Splenomegaly.
Thrombocytopenia and leucopenia.
Secondary to portal hypertension.

Bardet-Biedl Syndrome

Autosomal recessive.
Obesity.
Polydactyly.
Hypogenitalism.

Mental retardation.
Progressive retinitis pigmentosa.

Barlow Syndrome

Atypical chest pain.
Commoner in women.
Late apical systolic murmur.
Preceding ejection click radiating to axilla.
Mitral valve infections and arrhythmias.
Often of little clinical importance.

Bartter Syndrome

Hyperplasia of renal juxta glomerular apparatus.
Hypokalaemic alkalosis.
Hyperaldosteronism.
Normal blood pressure.

Batten-Vogt Syndrome
(v. Batten's Disease.)

Battered Baby Syndrome
(Non Accidental Injury.)

Commoner than medical profession are prepared to accept.
Squalid homes.
Parents of low intelligence.
Parents themselves may have had violent and unloved childhood.
May be one child singled out amongst siblings who are treated normally.

Classical X-ray findings are fragments separated from metaphyses and separation of periosteum due to subperiosteal bleeding.
Fractures of ribs and clavicles.
Death from subdural haematoma from violent shaking.

Baumgarten Syndrome
(v. Cruveilhier-Baumgarten Syndrome.)

Becker's Syndrome
(v. Becker's Muscular Dystrophy.)

Beckwith-Wiedman Syndrome
(Beckwith Syndrome.)

Thought to be autosomal dominant.
Exophthalmos, macroglossia and gigantism.
Grooved ears.
Umbilical abnormalities; small hernia to omphalocele.
Large kidneys and adrenals due to abnormal rate of growth.
Occasionally Wilms tumour of kidney.
Hypoglycaemia from abnormally large Islets of Langerhans.

Benedikt's Syndrome

Severe cerebellar signs on side opposite to 3rd nerve palsy.
Due to paramedian midbrain vascular lesion.

Bernard-Soulier Syndrome

Inherited disorder of platelet function.
Glycoprotein deficiency in platelet membrane.
Platelets large and morphologically abnormal.
Associated with severe bleeding diseases.

Bland-White-Garland Syndrome

Anomalous origin of left coronary artery from pulmonary artery.
Distal distribution normal.
Normal right coronary.
Angina pectoris and myocardial infarction in children.

Blind Loop Syndrome

Commonest in excessively long afferent loop after gastrectomy or gastroenterostomy.
Small bowel normally sterile.
Stasis results in bacterial colonisation.
Bile acids become deconjugated.
Steatorrhoea results.
Bacteria utilise Vitamin B12, thus impairing absorption.
Anaemia ensues.

Bloom's Syndrome

Chromosomal disorder.
Stunted growth.
Facial erythema.
Susceptible to leukaemia in second and third decades.

Blue Diaper Syndrome

Malabsorption of tryptophan from small intestine.
Tryptophane is converted to indoles.
Indoles excreted in the urine.

Boerhaave Syndrome

Strangulation of paraoesophageal hernia.
Spontaneous oesophageal perforation.
Presents acutely.
Life threatening.

Bonnevie-Ullrich Syndrome

Congenital lymphoedema of the extremities.
Webbing of neck.
Nail dystrophy.
Skin laxity.
Short stature.
Severe cardiac and renal anomalies.

Brandt's Syndrome

Steatorrhoea.
Alopecia.
Paronychia, perianal and perioral pustules.

Briquet's Syndrome
(Hypochondriasis.)

Involuntary physical complaints for which no physical cause is found. c.f. hysteria.

Demand medical attention and investigation.
Symptoms usually vague though described in dramatic terms.
Dyspnoea and dysphonia.
May follow current health trend.
Usually women.
Sexual and gynaecological symptoms common.

Brissaud-Sicard Syndrome

Facial hemi-spasm.
Contralateral hemiplegia.

Brock Syndrome
(Middle Lobe Syndrome.)

Recurrent chest infections.
Due to middle lobe collapse.
Due to compression middle lobe bronchus by enlarged lymph node.

Brown-Sequard Syndrome

One sided spinal cord compression.
A band of hyperaesthesia on the same side.
Below this - signs of an upper motor neurone lesion and loss of proprioceptive sensation.
On the other side - loss of pain, heat and cold sensation.
Unusual in pure form.
Incomplete form usually due to cervical disc protrusion.
May occur in multiple sclerosis.

Buchanan's Syndrome

Single artery supplying both pulmonary and systemic systems.
Arises from base of heart.
Cyanosed from birth.

Budd-Chiari Syndrome

Obstruction to hepatic venous outflow.
Causes include congenital malformation, thrombosis in polycythaemia vera, oral contraceptives, pressure from hepatic, renal or adrenal tumours.
Also in constrictive pericarditis or right ventricular failure.
Many cases show no obvious cause.
Hepatomegaly and ascites.
Caudate lobe may be spared by direct venous connections with inferior vena cava.
May cause death or cirrhosis or may recover completely.

Burning Feet Syndrome

Painful sensory neuropathy in the elderly.
Inadequate diet results in Vitamin B deficiency.
Pain in feet especially in bed at night.
Responds to Vitamin B complex.

Bywaters Syndrome
(v. Crush Syndrome.)

Cantrell's Syndrome

Midline, supraumbilical abdominal wall defect.

Defect in lower sternum.
Defect in anterior diaphragm.
Pericardial defect.
Ectopia cordis.
Ventricular septal defects.
May also have Fallot tetralogy.
Frequently fatal.

Capgras Syndrome

Most commonly found in schizophrenia.
May also occur in dementia.
Patient claims that people are their doubles, not truly themselves.

Caplan's Syndrome

Rheumatoid arthritis in miners with coal workers' pneumoconiosis.
Characteristic round fibrotic pulmonary nodules.

Carcinoid Syndrome

Carcinoid tumour (argentaffinoma).
Usually appendix, bowel or stomach.
Flushing.
Diarrhoea, may be severe.
Labile blood pressure.
Cardiac arrhythmias.
Pulmonary stenosis or tricuspid incompetence.
Bronchospasm.
Handling tumour exacerbates symptoms.
Large quantities 5-hydroxytryptophane in urine.

Carini's Syndrome

Shedding outer layers of dermis.
Produces "alligator baby".

Carpal Tunnel Syndrome

Median nerve compression at wrist beneath flexor retinaculum.
Middle aged women particularly.
Weakness and wasting small muscles of thumb.
Often bilateral.
Pain, numbness and paraesthesiae in distribution of median nerve.
Predisposing factors include vibrating tools, female hormonal imbalance, myxoedema, acromegaly, diabetes mellitus and rheumatoid arthritis.

Cervical Rib Syndrome
(Scalenus Anticus Syndrome. Naffziger Syndrome. Adson's Syndrome.)

Compression of C8 and T1 nerve roots.
Commonest in adolescent females with long necks.
Tingling and numbness along ulnar border of forearm.
Wasting thenar muscles.
In severe cases, wasting all intrinsic muscles of the hand.

Cestan-Chenais Syndrome

Tumour in pontobulbar region.
Or occlusion vertebral artery below posterior inferior cerebellar artery.

Ipsilateral soft palate and vocal cord paralysis.
Contralateral hemiplegia.
Sensory loss.
Ataxia.

Charcot-Marie-Tooth Syndrome
(Peroneal Muscular Atrophy.)

Demyelinating neurological disorder.
Motor and sensory.
Distal motor weakness.
Reduced or absent reflexes.
Affects particularly the peroneal muscle group.
May appear in childhood.
Normal life span.

Chediak-Higashi Syndrome

Very rare, autosomal recessive disorder.
Also found in mice, cattle and mink.
Partial oculocutaneous albinism with photophobia.
Abnormal white cells.
Enlarged liver and spleen.
Lymphadenopathy.
Changes in bone, lungs, heart and skin.
Prone to infection.
Most die in childhood from infection or haemorrhage.

Chiari-Frommel Syndrome
(Forbes-Albright Syndrome. Galactorrhoea.)

Lactation without suckling after pregnancy.

Due to excessive prolactin production by pituitary adenoma.
Amenorrhoea.
Uterine atrophy.

Churg-Strauss Syndrome
(Allergic Granulomatous Angiitis.)

Multisystem vasculitis.
Necrotising vasculitis of the gut, pulmonary and splenic vessels.
Associated with eosinophilic infiltration and granuloma formation.
Aneurysmal dilatations.
Multiple organ infarcts due to aneurysmal rupture, thrombosis or bleeding.
Bronchial asthma may occur.

Claude's Syndrome

A lesion involving red nucleus.
Ipsilateral oculomotor paralysis.
Contralateral ataxia and hemichorea.

Clumsy Child Syndrome

Poor motor skills.
Learning difficulties.
Thought due to subclinical brain damage from hypoxia or other birth injuries.
Phenobarbitone also in infancy.

Coalition Syndrome
(Peroneal Spastic Flat Foot.)

Flat foot may not be obvious.
Pain lateral side of foot.
Pain in peroneal tendons on passive inversion.
Bony, cartilaginous or fibrous coalition between calcaneus and navicular or talus and calcaneus.
May remain asymptomatic.

Cockayne Syndrome

Autosomal recessive enzyme disorder.
Abnormality in DNA repair may make cancer prone.
Normal at birth.
Appears at 6 - 12 months.
Physical retardation.
Severe dwarfism.
Wizened appearance.
Cerebral atrophy and demyelination.
Mental retardation.
Skin actinic sensitivity.
Cataracts.
Retinal and optic atrophy.
Sensori-neural deafness.
Atherosclerosis and osteoporosis.

Coffin-Lowry Syndrome
(Coffin Syndrome.)

Hereditary recessive X linked disorder.
Mental retardation.

Generalised hypotonia.
Short stature.
Square foreheads with widely separated eyes.
Tapered fingers.
Deafness.

Cogan's Syndrome

Acute onset in middle age.
Tinnitus, vertigo and deafness.
Ocular interstitial keratitis.
Aortitis.
Aortic valvular disease.
Raised serum immunoglobulins.

Collet-Sicard Syndrome

Damage to last four cranial nerves.
Usually due to extracranial lesion (cf. Vernet's syndrome).

Conn's Syndrome
(Primary Aldersteronism.)

Primary cause is benign tumour of adrenal glomerulosa cells.
High blood level of aldosterone.
Hypertension due to salt and water retention, producing intravascular volume expansion.
Hypokalaemia.
Alkalosis.
Weakness.
Polyuria and thirst.
Muscle cramps.

Cardiac arrhythmias.
Glycosuria.

Conradi-Hunerman Syndrome

Teratogenic effects of warfarin therapy in first trimester.
Saddle nose due to nasal hypoplasia.
Frontal bossing.
Short stature.
Stippled epiphyses.
Optic atrophy and cataracts.
Mental retardation and contractures.

Cornelia de Lange Syndrome
(Brachmann de Lange Syndrome. Amsterdam Dwarfism.)

Mental retardation.
Short stature.
Microcephaly.
Deformities of hands and arms with Simian creases.
Normal legs but webbing between 2nd and 3rd toes.
Long upper lip with trianglar mouth.
Cardiac abnormalities.
Convulsions and hypertonia.
Hirsutism with synophrys.
Susceptible to infection.
Few reach old age.

Coroli Syndrome

Cystic dilatation of intrahepatic ducts.
Gall stones.

Cholangitis.
Increased incidence of cholangiocarcinoma.

Costen's Syndrome

Pain in temperomandibular joint.
Normally occurs due to malocclusion in edentulous.
May also be psychological in origin.
Feature of depression.

Cotard's Syndrome

Nihilistic delusions (denies his own existence).
May request burial, deluded he is a corpse.
Associated with depression, alcoholism, neurosyphilis.

Couvade Syndrome

Symptoms suffered by fathers-to-be during wife's childbearing.
Backache.
Abdominal pain.
Weight gain.
Toothache.

CREST Syndrome

Connective tissue disorder.
C - calcinosis circumscripta.
R - Raynaud's phenomenon.
E - (o)esophageal disease.
S - sclerodactyly.
T - telangiectasia.
Specific antinuclear antibody present in serum.

Cri-du-Chat Syndrome

Rare congenital disorder.
Absent short arm of chromosome 5.
M : F :: 1 : 2
Mental retardation with characteristic wailing cry.
Abnormal skin patterns on palms and soles.
Microcephaly.
Facial abnormalities.
Cardiac malformations.
Failure to thrive.

Crigler-Najjar Syndrome
(Congenital Hyperbilirubinaemia.)

Infants deficient in glucuronyl transferase in the liver.
Essential to bilirubin metabolism.
Large accumulations of bilirubin in brain.
Severe, permanent central nervous system damage.
Kernicterus (damage to basal ganglia).
Convulsions, coma, opisthotonus, deafness, mental retardation.
Usually early death; few survive to adulthood.

Cronkhite-Canada Syndrome

Polyposis generalised throughout gastro-intestinal tract.
Diarrhoea.
Steatorrhoea.
Alopecia.
Nail dystrophy.
Skin hyperpigmentation.
Brown macules face and limbs.

Crouzon's Syndrome
(Crouzon's Disease. Craniofacial Dysostosis.)

Cranio-facial malformations.
Premature fusion of coronal, sagittal and sometimes lambdoid skull sutures.
Frontal bones poorly developed.
Premature fusion of metopic suture produces triangular shaped head (trigonocephaly).
Anteroposterior cranial diameter reduced.
Brain development enlarges transverse diameter.
Proptosis due to shallow orbits.
Corneal ulceration.
Hypertelorism.
Underdeveloped maxilla.

Crush Syndrome
(Bywaters Syndrome.)

Renal failure following severe crush injury to a limb (usually leg).
Hypovolaemia due to fluid loss into damaged muscles.
Free myoglobin released into the circulation.
Causes vasoconstriction, renal ischaemia and tubular necrosis.

Cruveilhier-Baumgarten Syndrome

Portal venous obstruction.
Large shunt via umbilical vein.
Venous bruit in midline.

Cubital Tunnel Syndrome

Ulnar nerve compression between two heads of flexor carpi ulnaris.
Pain in ulnar distribution in forearm and hand.

Curtis-Fitz-Hugh Syndrome

Young women.
Right upper quadrant pain and peritonitis.
No clinical or radiological evidence of gall stones or cholecystitis.
Localised perihepatitis caused by Chlamydia Trachomatis infection.
May also have chlamydial genital tract infection.

Cushing's Syndrome

Due to primary or secondary adrenal cortical overactivity.
M : F :: 1 : 4 - except in ectopic cases.
Primary adrenal cortical tumour.
Secondary to pituitary tumour (Cushing's Disease).
May be iatrogenic from hormone therapy with ACTH or corticosteroids.
May result from ectopic ACTH production by non endocrine tumours e.g. carcinoma of bronchus.
Obesity with purple striae and "buffalo hump".
Muscle wasting.
Florid appearance with "moon" face.
Hypertension.
Skin atrophy with haemorrhages.
Osteoporosis.
Diabetes mellitus.

Suppressed ovulation with amenorrhoea.
Hirsutism and acne.
Remission of symptoms is possible if cause of excess cortisol production is removed.
Structural changes to heart, blood vessels, kidneys and bone likely to remain.

da Costa Syndrome
(Effort Syndrome. Soldier's Heart. Cardiac Neurosis.)

Palpitations.
Precordial pain.
Sense of fatigue.
Panic attacks.
No structural cardiac abnormality.

Dandy-Walker Syndrome

Hypoplastic cerebellum.
Congenital occlusion foramina (Magendie and Luschka) to fourth ventricle.
Enlarged posterior fossa.
Hydrocephalus with gross distension of fourth ventricle.

de Clerambault's Syndrome
(Erotomania.)

Usually single woman.
Deluded someone of higher social status, even famous, is in love with her.

Degos's Syndrome
(Degos Disease)

Skin lesions related to intestinal disease.
Skin papules due to endovasculitis with atrophic, white centres.
Similar lesions in gastro-intestinal tract.
Multiple intestinal infarcts.
Abdominal cramps and vomiting.
Enteritis with haemorrhage and perforation.
May also involve nervous system.
Often fatal.

de Grouchy's Syndrome

Disorder of chromosome 18.
Two types, 18q and 18p, both mentally retarded.
18q - "carp mouth", abnormal ears and tapering fingers.
18p - eye, ear and CNS abnormalities.

Dejerine-Roussy Syndrome
(Thalamic syndrome.)

Due to vascular lesion in posterior thalamus.
Resulting disabilities are unilateral.
Loss of sensation.
Inability to recognise objects.
Varying degree of paralysis.
Incoordination.
Severe pain induced by stimuli above a certain strength.
Choreoathetoid movements of arm and leg.

Del Castillo Syndrome
(Testicular Dysgenesis.)

Hypogonadism in otherwise normal looking males.
Absent germinal epithelium.
Sterility.
Androgen replacement ineffective.

Diamond-Blackfan Syndrome
(Blackfan-Diamond Syndrome. Erythrogenesis Imperfecta.)

Inherited defect in erythroid production.
Increasing pallor first few months of life.
Both sexes - milder form in boys.
No haemorrhagic signs.
Normocytic, normochromic anaemia.
Dwarfism but normal intelligence.
Repeated blood transfusions may lead to haemosiderosis, cirrhosis, portal hypertension and hypersplenism.

Di George Syndrome
(Thymic Aplasia.)

Congenital absence of thymus and parathyroid glands.
May have aortic arch anomaly.
Hypocalcaemia.
Tetany in the newborn.
Hypertelorism.
Predisposed to infection.
Few survive.

Down Syndrome
(Down's Syndrome. Mongolism. Trisomy 21.)

Congenital due to extra chromosome 21.
Broad face on short neck.
Brachycephaly (short skull).
Slanting eyes with inner epicanthic fold.
Large tongue.
Characteristic skin patterns on palms (single transverse crease) and soles.
Mental retardation but quiet personalities with love of music.
40% have some cardiac or renal malformation.
Liable to develop acute leukaemia.
Females are capable of childbearing; 50% offspring likely to be Downs.
Roughly 1:800 live births but 1:40 in mothers over 40.
Reduced life expectancy due to accelerated ageing processes.
Features less marked in mosaics where not all cell lines are affected by trisomy.

Dresbach's Syndrome
(Hereditary Elliptocytosis.)

Inherited autosomal dominant.
Haemolysis of elliptical shaped erythrocytes.
Anaemia.
Leg ulcers.
Maxillofacial abnormalities.

Dressler's Syndrome
(Post Myocardial Infarct Syndrome.)

Fever, pericarditis and pleurisy.
Weeks or months after infarct.
Autoimmune reaction to dead myocardium.
Often subsides after few days.

Duane's Retraction Syndrome

Retraction of ocular globe on attempted adduction.
20% bilateral.
Perceptive deafness.
Speech disorder.

Dubin-Johnson Syndrome
(Congenital Hyperbilirubinaemia.)

Autosomal recessive disorder of bilirubin metabolism.
Malaise.
Chronic, intermittent mild jaundice.
Raised serum bilirubin (conjugated - c.f. Gilbert's syndrome).
Bile in urine.
Intracellular brown pigment on biopsy (c.f. Gilbert's syndrome).
Excellent prognosis.

Dumping Syndrome
(Post Gastrectomy Syndrome.)

Drowsiness, weakness and nausea after a meal.
Flushing.
Palpitations.
Particularly after hot sweet food.
Tends to improve.

Dysmnesic Syndrome

Chronic memory impairment without significant intellectual or personality change (cf. dementia).

Eagle-Barrett Syndrome
(v. Prune Belly Syndrome.)

Eaton-Lambert Syndrome
(Lambert-Eaton Myasthenic Syndrome. LEMS.)

Form of myasthenic weakness.
Proximal muscles especially legs.
Tendon reflexes diminished at rest, increased on exercise.
Initial muscle weakness is overcome by increasing strength as muscle contracts only to return if contraction is maintained.
Dry throat.
Paraneoplastic syndrome.
Associated with small cell carcinoma of lung.

Ebstein's Anomaly Syndrome

Congenital disorder of tricuspid valve.
Anterior cusp is grossly enlarged.
Posterior and septal cusps arise near apex of right ventricle.
Part of right ventricle thus incorporated into right atrium.
Tricuspid incompetence.
Dyspnoea on exertion.
Variable cyanosis.
Loud first heart sound with short systolic murmur.
Death from right heart failure.

Edwards's Syndrome
(Trisomy 18.)

Due to extra chromosome 18.
Commoner in infants born to mothers over 35.
Infants rarely survive more than few months.
Mental and growth retardation.
Long narrow skull with prominent occiput.
Congenital heart defects.
Cleft lip and palate.
Webbed neck with malformed, malimplanted ears.
Receding chin (micrognathia).
Flexion finger deformities.
"Rocker bottom" feet.
Differentiation from Patau's syndrome may be difficult.

Ehlers-Danlos Syndrome
(Cutis Hyperelastica.)

Rare hereditary disorder.
Velvety, fragile, elastic skin.
Lax joints frequently dislocating.
Bruise readily due to capillary fragility.
May lead to aortic dilatation and aneurysm in childhood.

Eisenmenger Syndrome

Pulmonary hypertension.
Ventricular or atrial septal defect or patent ductus arteriosus.
Right to left (reverse) shunt.
Pulmonary hypertension.
Gross cardiomegaly.

Symptoms in childhood.
Failure to thrive.
Lethargy.
Respiratory infections.
Polycythaemia.
Pulmonary infarction.
Closure of septal defect may be contraindicated.

Ekbom Syndrome
(v. Restless Legs Syndrome.)

Ellis-van Creveld Syndrome
(Chondroectodermal Dysplasia.)

Recessive, hereditary, congenital disorder.
Cardiac defects, commonly atrial septal.
Polydactyly.
Defective teeth and nails.
Dwarfism.
Genu valgum.

Engelmann's Syndrome
(Progressive Diaphysial Dysplasia. Camurati's Disease.)

Recessive, hereditary disorder of bone.
Begins in childhood.
"Tired legs".
Thickening of shafts of long bones and vault of skull.
Painless.
Tall with waddling gait.
Weak and easily fatigued.

X-rays show fusiform widening and sclerosis of shafts of long bones, sometimes skull.

Epstein Syndrome
(v. Nephrotic Syndrome.)

Fanconi Syndrome
(de Toni-Fanconi Syndrome. Cystinosis.)

Hereditary autosomal recessive.
May be acquired.
Failure to thrive, thirst, polyuria, constipation.
Renal tubular failure.
Widespread cystine crystal deposits throughout reticulo-endothelial system.
Hypokalaemia.
Deformities due to rickets.
Osteomalacia.
Nephrocalcinosis and renal stone formation.

Favre-Goldmann Syndrome

Rare autosomal recessive disorder.
Nightblindness in children.
Retinal pigmentary changes.

Felty's Syndrome

Rheumatoid arthritis.
Long standing but inactive cases.
Splenomegaly.
Neutropenia.

Anaemia.
Thrombocytopaenia.
Weight loss.
Skin pigmentation.
Leg ulcers.

Fisher Syndrome

Ophthalmoplegia.
Ataxia.
Loss of tendon reflexes.
Usually recovers completely.

Foetal Alcohol Syndrome

Infants of alcoholic mothers.
Small foetus.
Small head with facial deformities.
Joint defects in hands and feet.
Cleft palate.
Heart defects.
Mental retardation.

Forbes-Albright Syndrome
(Chiari-Frommel Syndrome. Galactorrhoea.)

Lactation without suckling after pregnancy.
Due to excessive prolactin production by pituitary.

Foster-Kennedy Syndrome

Optic atrophy one eye due to direct pressure on the optic nerve.

Papilloedema in other eye due to raised intracranial pressure.
Tumours of inferior surface of frontal lobe of cerebrum.
Meningioma sphenoidal ridge or olfactory groove.

Foville's Syndrome

Caused by lesion in pons.
Ipsilateral VIth nerve palsy.
Gaze palsy.
Facial palsy.
Facial analgesia.
Horner's syndrome.
Deafness.
Contralateral spastic paralysis.

Fragile X Syndrome

Abnormally fragile portion of X chromosome.
Males with fragile X will develop mental retardation.
One third females with fragile X will develop mental retardation.
All females with fragile X stand 50/50 chance of passing on defect.

Francheschetti-Klein Syndrome
(Treacher-Collins Syndrome. Mandibulofacial Dysostosis.)

Rare, dominant hereditary genetic disorder.
Underdeveloped facial bones and lower jaw.
Hypertelorism.
Malformation of lower eyelid.
No eyelashes.
No external auditory canal.

Deafness.
Normal intelligence.

Fregoli Syndrome

Patient thinks those he meets are identical with a person he knows well.
Believes him to be his persecutor.

Frey's Syndrome

Complication of parotidectomy.
Discomfort, sweating and erythema over parotid region on eating.
Severed ends of secretomotor parasympathetic fibres (formerly involved in salivation) grow into skin.
Usually resolves spontaneously in six months.

Frohlich's Syndrome
(Adiposogenital Dystrophy.)

Metabolic disorder.
Mostly boys.
Usually due to hypothalamic tumour (craniopharyngioma), encephalitis or trauma.
Increased appetite leading to obesity.
Growth retardation.
Reduced gonadotrophic hormone secretion.
Underdeveloped genitals.
Poor vision due to optic nerve pressure by tumour.

Froin's Syndrome

Lumbar puncture findings in spinal cord compression.

Xanthochromia.
Grossly raised protein in CSF.
Normal cell count.

Ganser Syndrome
(Hysterical Pseudodementia.)

Absurd answers given to simple questions.
Inconsistent behaviour.
Visual hallucinatory experiences.
Clouding of consciousness.
May be seen in schizophrenia.
Also in prisoners awaiting trial.

Gardner's Syndrome

Polyposis coli.
Sebaceous cysts.
Osteomata face and skull.
Desmoid tumours.
Multiple fibromata.
Rarely benign gastric and duodenal polyps.
Periampullary carcinoma may occur.

Gerstmann's Syndrome

Agraphia.
Acalculia.
Finger agnosia.
Right/left disorientation.
Usually lesion in region of angular gyrus in dominant parietal lobe.

Gerstmann-Straussler Syndrome

Rare familial and transmissable viral infection.
Resembles CJD but no myoclonus and more prominent spasticity.
Brain shows amyloid plaques.

Gilbert's Syndrome
(Congenital Hyperbilirubinaemia.)

Autosomal dominant disorder of bilirubin metabolism.
First recognised usually in adolescence - 2nd and 3rd decades.
Often symptomless.
Episodic malaise, anorexia and mild jaundice.
Jaundice increases on fasting.
Raised serum bilirubin (unconjugated - c.f. Dubin-Johnson syndrome).
Acholuric.
Liver biopsy normal (c.f. Dubin-Johnson syndrome).
May arise as benign cause of post-anaesthetic jaundice.
Prognosis excellent.
Only danger is misdiagnosis for some more serious liver complaint.

Gilles de la Tourette's Syndrome
(v. Tourette's Syndrome.)

Goldenhar Syndrome
(Goldenhar-Gorlin Syndrome.
Oculoauricular Vertebral Syndrome.)

Accurate diagnosis may be difficult.
Deafness due to middle and external ear deformities.

Facial asymmetry, increasingly obvious in early years.
Cleft palate.
Hypoplasia upper and lower jaws.
Microtia.
Vertebral abnormalities.
Scoliosis.
Cardiac abnormalities, commonly ventricular septal defect.
Strabismus.
Optic nerve and macular hypoplasia.

Goodpasture's Syndrome

Rare form of glomerulonephritis.
Haemoptysis due to acute haemorrhagic pneumonitis.
Complication of autoimmune vascular disease such as periarteritis nodosa.

Good's Syndrome

Thymoma in conjunction with agammaglobulinaemia.
Impaired immunity to fungal, viral and pyogenic infections.

Gordon's Syndrome

Hypertension.
Increased extracellular fluid volume.
Low aldosterone levels.
Hyperkalaemia.
Growth retardation.
Intermittent paralysis.
All reversed by sodium restriction.

Gorlin's Syndrome

Multiple basal cell carcinomas.
Mandibular cysts.
Mesenteric cysts.
Scoliosis.
Palmar and plantar pits.

Gradenigo Syndrome

Rare complication of middle ear infection.
Caused by infection of apex of petrous temporal bone over which VIth nerve runs.
Diplopia from lateral rectus palsy.
Trigeminal pain.
Evidence of middle ear infection.

Grey Baby Syndrome

Follows chloramphenicol therapy in premature and newborn infants.
Inadequate conjugation of chloramphenicol in the infant liver.
Peripheral circulatory collapse.
Abdominal distension.
Diarrhoea and vomiting.
Frequently fatal.

Gronblad-Strandberg Syndrome
(Pseudoxanthoma Elasticum.)

Recessive inherited disorder of elastic tissue.
Loss of skin elasticity, skin hanging loosely.
Thickening of exposed skin with yellow plaques.

Axilla, groins and abdomen also affected.
Poor peripheral circulation.
Spontaneous haemorrhages.
Brown/black retinal streaks.
Visual impairment.

Guillain-Barre Syndrome
(Acute Infective Polyneuritis.)

Demyelinating polyneuropathy.
Acute post inflammatory, one to four weeks after viral infection.
Autoimmune reaction attacks the myelin sheath of motor nerves.
Proximal muscular weakness may progress to respiratory distress.
Bilateral facial weakness.
Loss of reflexes.
Peripheral paraesthesiae but few sensory complications.
Spontaneous remission within weeks.

Haemolytic-Uraemic Syndrome

Commoner in infants and children than adults.
Usually follows an acute febrile illness.
Has been described as following vaccination.
Renal changes include thrombi in glomerular tufts and cortical necrosis.
Thrombocytopenia.
Red cell destruction in diseased small vessels (microangiopathic).
Haemolytic anaemia.

Haglund's Syndrome

Painful bursa along Achilles tendon.
Caused by rigid low backed shoes.

Hallerman-Streiff-Francoise Syndrome

All signs of premature ageing (progeria).
Dwarfism.
Microphthalmia.
Cataracts.
Micrognathia.
Psychomotor retardation.

Hallgren's Syndrome

Usher's syndrome with additional mental instability and retardation.

Hand-Foot Syndrome

Symmetrical painful swelling of fingers and feet.
Infarction of small blood vessels to bone in sickle cell disease.
X-rays show severe bone destruction and periosteal reaction.

Heerfordt's Syndrome

Sarcoidosis.
Uveitis.
Salivary gland enlargement.
Lachrymal gland enlargement.

Hepato-renal Syndrome

Progressive renal failure occurring with advanced liver disease.
May be terminal stage of hepatic failure.
Combination of hepatic and renal failure as disease entity is disputed.

Renal blood flow is reduced due to arteriolar vasoconstriction in renal cortex.
Renal shutdown resulting from shock is common in the severely jaundiced.
Less than 5% survive without liver transplant.
Renal failure is reversed after liver transplant.

Holmes-Adie Syndrome

Absent tendon reflexes on same side as Adie pupil.
- Pupil tonically dilated but may be found constricted.
- Dilates slowly in the dark.
- Constriction to light or accommodation is slow.
- Varies in size but never reacts promptly.
- Frequently unilateral (anisocoria).
- Hypersensitive reaction to weak cholinergic drug instillation.

Sweating disorder.
Postural hypotension.

Holt-Oram Syndrome

Autosomal dominant.
Atrial septal defects.
Short forearms.
Triphalangeal thumbs.

Horner's Syndrome

Impaired cervical sympathetic nerve supply.
Ptosis.
Enophthalmos.
Miosis.
Flushed facial skin.

Anhydrosis.
Blocked nostril.

Howell-Evans Syndrome
(Palmoplantar Keratoderma.)

Dominant inherited trait.
Benign thickening skin of palms and soles (tylosis).

Hungry Bones Syndrome

Hypocalcaemia and tetany with magnesium depletion.
Follows removal of parathyroid adenoma or total parathyroidectomy for severe hyperparathyroidism with bone invovement.

Hunter's Syndrome
(Gargoylism.)

Hereditary, recessive X-linked disorder.
Deficiency of enzyme essential in mucopolysaccharide metabolism.
Males only.
Unaffected sister at risk of having affected son.
Onset in first three years.
Mental retardation.
No clouding of the cornea.
Deafness.
Dwarfism.
Hirsutism and claw hands.
Usually die from respiratory infections before early adulthood.
A milder variety may survive to middle age.

Hunt's Syndrome

Pyridoxine deficiency.
Intractable neonatal fits.
Fatal without treatment.

Hurler's Syndrome
(Gargoylism)

Autosomal, recessive, genetic disorder of mucopolysaccharide metabolism.
Onset in infancy or early childhood in either sex.
Unaffected girl unlikely to have affected child unless by a close relative carrying the mutant gene.
Mental retardation.
Hirsutism.
Deafness.
Corneal clouding.
Enlarged liver and spleen.
Hunch backed dwarf with short limbs and clawed hands.
Large head with prominent brows and poorly formed teeth.
Usually die from heart failure during adolescence.

Hutchinson-Gilford Syndrome
(Infant Progeria.)

Premature ageing appearing in early childhood.
Develop physical attributes of old age.
Susceptible to diseases of old age.
CNS is exempt.
No senility.
Signs appear at about one year.
May appear 60 years old at age 10.

Underdeveloped external genitalia.
Atherosclerosis and heart disease by age 10.
Rarely reach age of 30 years.

Hyperprolactinaemia Syndrome

Pituitary prolactinoma.
Also side effects of any drug that antagonises dopamine.
Galactorrhoea in both sexes.
Oligomenorrhoea or amenorrhoea in women.
Loss of libido and impotence in men.
High blood levels of prolactin indicates presence of prolactinoma.

Irritable Bowel Syndrome
(Spastic Colon.)

Commoner in nervous, anxious, conscientious personalities.
Most common in women 20 to 40 years of age.
Has no organic cause.
Constipation.
Watery diarrhoea.
Abdominal discomfort.
Spasmodic pain, mainly in left or right iliac fossa.

Ivemark Syndrome
(Congenital Asplenia.)

Absent spleen.
Cyanotic heart disease.
Bowel malrotation and situs inversus.
Death from overwhelming infection.

Jaccoud's Syndrome

Severe deformities, particularly hands and feet, resembling rheumatoid arthritis.
Rare permanent residual complication of acute rheumatic fever.
May also follow joint involvement in systemic lupus erythematosus.

Jansen's Syndrome
(Congenital Metaphyseal Dysostosis.)

Dwarfism.
Mental retardation.
Widely spaced exophthalmic eyes.
Funnel chest.
Usually die in childhood.

Job's Syndrome

Disease of girls with red hair.
Clinically resembles chronic granulomatous disease.
Impaired phagocytosis due probably to enzyme deficiency.
Predisposes to chronic pyogenic infections.

Jones-Nevin Syndrome
(Subacute Spongiform Encephalopathy.)

Disease of adults aged 50 to 70 years.
Rapidly progressive dementia.
Myoclonic jerking.
May be a variant of Creutzfeldt-Jakob Disease.

Kallmann's Syndrome

Congenital hypothalamic defect.
Hypogonadism due to deficient gonadotrophin production.
Underdeveloped penis.
Failure to undergo puberty.
Anosmia.

Kanner's Syndrome

Autism.

Kartagener's Syndrome

Bronchiectasis.
Sinusitis.
Transposition of the viscera.

Kasabach-Merritt Syndrome

Sudden increase in size of cavernous haemangioma.
Associated development of thrombocytopenia due to platelet sequestration in the tumour.
May prove fatal.

Kast's Syndrome
(v. Maffucci's Syndrome.)

Kawasaki Syndrome
(Mucocutaneous Lymph Node Syndrome.)

Usually children under 5 years.

Cause unknown.
Acute inflammatory disease.
Fever.
Conjuctival congestion.
Cervical lymphadenopathy.
Skin rash with reddening of palms and soles.
One fifth develop heart disease due to coronary artery damage.

Kearns-Sayre Syndrome

Progressive ophthalmoplegia.
Ptosis.
Heart block (sudden death).
Usually presents before 20 years.
Short stature.
Cerebellar ataxia.
Deafness.
Mental retardation.
Pigmentary retinopathy.

Kiloh-Nevin Syndrome

Weakness long flexors of thumb and index finger.
Lesion of anterior interosseous nerve.

Kleine-Levin Syndrome

Young males.
May follow infective illness.
Recurrent periods of severe somnolence and deep sleep.
May last days or weeks at a time.
May have visual or auditory hallucinations if woken forcibly.

Associated with gross eating when awake.
Does not complain of hunger if food not provided.

Klinefelter's Syndrome

Chromosome disorder in 1:1000 males.
More common with mother over 35 years.
Extra X chromosome (XXY) giving total of 47.
May also be XXXY, XXXXY or XXYY.
Eunuchoid body.
Aspermic with small undescended testes lacking normal sensation.
Enlarged breasts and buttocks.
Breast tumours common.
Underdeveloped external genitalia.
Tall with long legs.
Increased incidence of diabetes mellitus and goitre.
Lesser features occur in mosaics where not all cell lines are
    not involved.
Mental retardation particularly in XXXY.

Klippel-Feil Syndrome

M : F :: 2 : 3.
Short webbed neck.
Low hair line over back of neck.
Fused cervical or thoracic vertebrae.
Limitation of movement.
Rarely may also include -
    Horse shoe kidneys.
    Squint.
    Cleft palate.
    Deafness.

Ventricular septal defects.
Neuroblastoma.

Klippel-Trenaunay Syndrome
(Klippel-Trenaunay-Weber Syndrome.)

Haemangioma - port wine stain of an extremity.
Formation of AV fistulae.
Varicose veins.
Macrosomia with bone and soft tissue hypertrophy.
Hemihypertrophy.
Changes may remain stationary after growth ceases.

Kluver-Bucy Syndrome

Psychic blindness (inability to identify friends and relatives).
Memory loss.
Over eating.
Heightened sexual activity.
Altered emotional responses.
Usually due to damage to medial temporal lobe.

Korsakoff's Syndrome
(Korsakoff Psychosis.)

Usually due to thiamine deficiency.
Usually result of severe, chronic alcoholism.
Also may follow severe head injury.
Normal consciousness and perception.
Severe amnesia for recent events.
Memory may be restricted to few seconds only.
Confabulation - fabrication of memories compensating true memory loss.

Lambert's Syndrome
(Porcupine Man.)

Congenital hyperkeratosis.
Spares hands, face and genitalia.

Lambert-Eaton Myasthenic Syndrome
(LEMS. Eaton-Lambert Syndrome.)

Form of myasthenic weakness.
Proximal muscles especially pelvic and shoulder girdles.
Tendon reflexes diminished at rest, increased on exercise.
Repeated muscular activity leads to strength rather than weakness (cf. myasthenia gravis).
Dry throat.
Associated with small cell carcinoma of lung.

LAMB Syndrome

L - lentigenes.
A - atrial myxoma.
M - mucocutaneous myxoma.
B - blue naevi.

Larsen's Syndrome

Presents in infancy.
Marked joint laxity.
Dislocation of hip.
Unstable knees.
Radial head subluxation.
Spinal deformities.

Lawrence-Moon-Biedl Syndrome
(Lawrence-Moon Syndrome.)

Autosomal recessive disorder, possibly enzyme.
Mental retardation.
Retinitis pigmentosa.
Visual difficulties beginning with night blindness.
Ataxia progressing to spastic paraplegia.
Underdeveloped genitalia.
Obesity.
Polydactyly or syndactyly.

LEOPARD Syndrome
(Cardio-cutaneous Syndrome.)

Rare autosomal dominant.
May be present at birth.
Develops by five years old.
L - lentigines - dark brown spots over face and body, always small and unaffected by sunlight.
E - ECG conduction defect.
O - ocular hypertelorism
P - pulmonary stenosis - 50%.
A - abnormal genitalia - hypospadias, cryptorchidism.
R - retarded growth.
D - deafness - 25% have sensineural.

Leriche Syndrome

Arteriosclerosis aortic bifurcation.
Usually 40 to 50 year old.
Intermittent claudication in legs and buttocks.

Gluteal wasting.
May mimic sciatica.
Impotence in the male.
Absent or diminished femoral pulses.
Hyperlipidaemia common.

Lermoyez Syndrome

Episodic deafness and tinnitus lasting few days.
Followed by episodes of vertigo.
Followed by improvement in hearing.
(Sometimes called the reverse form of Meniere's disease.)

Lesch-Nyhan Syndrome

Recessive hereditary disorder of purine metabolism chiefly in brain cells.
X chromosome linked.
Predominantly males.
Detectable during pregnancy in women carriers.
Gout.
Choreoathetosis (muscular incoordination).
Severe mental retardation.
Aggressive behaviour including compulsive biting and self mutilation.

Levy-Roussy Syndrome
(Roussy-Levy Syndrome.)

Hereditary neurological defect.
Appears in early childhood.
Scoliosis.

Club foot.
Progressive lower limb muscular atrophy.
Loss of deep reflexes.
Walking and standing difficulties due to muscular incoordination.
Cerebellar signs usually mild.

Liddle's Sydrome

Familial.
Excessive sodium reabsorption from distal renal tubules.
Salt retention.
Hypokalaemia.
Hypertension.
Simulates primary aldosteronism but aldosterone is suppressed.

Locked In Syndrome

Mental function including cognition is preserved.
No voluntary movement except vertical eye and eyelid movement (blinking).

Loeffler's Syndrome

Pulmonary infiltration with eosinophilia.
Asthma.
Alveolar exudation and increased mucus secretion.
Transient condition associated with helminthic infections and brucellosis.

Louis-Bar Syndrome
(Ataxia-telangiectasia.)

Autosomal recessive.
May be due to chromosome 14 abnormalities.
Cerebellar incoordination with ataxia.
Second or third year of life.
Telangiectases begin to appear 3 to 7 years - conjunctiva, face, ears.
Choreic movements.
Immune system disorders, usually severe IgA deficiency.
Severe sino-respiratory infections.
Death may be from bronchiectasis.
May develop malignancy e.g. lymphosarcoma.

Lowe's Syndrome
(Oculo-cerebro-renal Syndrome.)

Inherited, recessive X linked disorder.
Males only.
Women carriers.
Congenital cataracts and glaucoma.
Squints and nystagmus.
Gradual renal tubular failure.
Renal failure by mid childhood.
Rickets and hypotonia.
Areflexia.
Intelligence may vary from normal to severely handicapped.

Lucey-Driscoll Syndrome

Neonatal jaundice.
Familial.
Caused by tranplacental spread of unidentified factor in maternal serum.

Lutembacher's Syndrome

Atrial septal defect with mitral stenosis.
Raised left atrial pressure.
Distended left atrium enlarges septal defect.
Shunting and pulmonary hypertension.

Luxury Perfusion Syndrome

Blood flow over and above metabolic needs (v. Robin Hood Syndrome).
Damaged cerebral tissue in region of tumour, trauma or infarct.
Due to localised loss of autoregulation.

MacLeod's Syndrome

Unilateral emphysema.
Damage occurs before aged 8 years.
Other lung unaffected.
May follow measles or tuberculosis.
Often asymptomatic.
Radiology - unilateral hypertranslucency with oligaemia.

Maffucci's Syndrome
(Kast's Syndrome.)

May run in families.
Cutaneous haemangiomata.
Endochondromatosis
From minimal changes to gross deformities.
May develop chondrosarcoma.

Mallory-Weiss Syndrome

Haematemesis.
Lacerations in mucosa of cardiac end of stomach.
Follows bout of violent vomiting.
Usually after alcoholic debauch.

Marchesani Syndrome
(v. Weill-Marchesani Syndrome.)

Marcus Gunn (Jaw Blinking) Syndrome

Accounts for 5% of congenital ptosis.
Move jaw to one side.
Ptotic lid retracts (wink) on other side.

Marfan's Syndrome
(Arachnodactyly.)

Hereditary disorder of connective tissue.
Tall with long, thin limbs.
Joint laxity or dislocation.
Long slender "spidery" fingers (arachnodactyly).
High arched palate.

Dislocation of optic lens, sometimes congenital.
Glaucoma and retinal detachment.
Cardiac abnormalities e.g. mitral valve prolapse and regurgitation.
Liability to rupture of dissecting aneurysm of aorta.
Death from cardiovascular problems - 1/3 by 32 years; 2/3 by 50 years.

Marie and Sanger-Brown Syndrome

Strongly hereditary.
Late onset.
Ataxia.
Brisk reflexes.
Severe spasticity lower limbs.
Optic atrophy.
Easily misdiagnosed as multiple sclerosis.

Maroteaux-Lamy Syndrome

Rare recessive, hereditary disorder of mucopolysaccharide metabolism.
Onset in early childhood.
Dwarfism.
Deafness.
Skeletal deformity.
Corneal opacities.
Hypertelorism.
Enlarged liver and spleen.
Normal intelligence.
Seldom survive beyond 20 years.

McCune-Albright Syndrome
(Fibrous Dysplasia.)

Rare congenital disorder of bone.
Cyst formation.
Long bones and pelvis replaced by fibrous tissue.
Often unilateral.
Pathological fractures.
Unilateral enlargement of facial bones and base of skull.
Cafe au lait spots on skin.
Precocious puberty especially in females.

Megacystitis Mega-Ureter Syndrome

More common in girls.
Chronic or recurring pyuria.
Bilateral ureteric dilatation.
Grossly distended, apparently insensitive bladder.
No evidence of bladder neck obstruction.

Meig's Syndrome

Benign ovarian tumour.
Similar appearance to uterine fibroid.
Whorled cut surface.
Ascites.
Pleural effusion, almost always right sided.

Meige's Syndrome

Blepharospasm, severe enough for loss of vision from permanently closed eyelids.

Torticollis.
Oromandibular dystonia.

Mendelsohn's Syndrome

Gastric acid reflux and aspiration during obstetric anaesthesia.
Mortality rate may be 25%.
Predisposing factors in pregnancy -
   delay in gastric emptying
   incompetent cardiac sphincter
   raised intra-abdominal pressure.

Menke's Syndrome
(Kinky Hair Syndrome.)

X-linked recessive disorder of copper metabolism in boys.
Copper deficiency due to impaired intestinal transport.
Presents with seizures in infancy.
Growth retardation.
Pale skin.
Changes in the hair.
Central nervous system degeneration.
Poor prognosis.
Death usually in second year.

Millard-Gubler Syndrome

Caused by lesion in the pons.
Ipsilateral VIth nerve palsy.
Eye on side of lesion cannot abduct.
Contralateral hemiplegia.

Miller-Fisher Syndrome

Acute onset after viral infection.
Ophthalmoplegia.
Ataxia.
Areflexia.
Pupillary paralysis.
Recovery within days.
Excellent prognosis.

Mirizzi's Syndrome
(Cholecysto-choledochal Fistula.)

Gall stone impacts in gall bladder neck.
Ulcerates into common duct.
Fistula formed between gall bladder and extrahepatic biliary tree.
Pain and jaundice.

Moebius' Syndrome

Agenesis motor ganglion cells in some cranial nerves.
Most commonly abducens and facial nerves.
Eye deviated medially with diplopia.
Facial palsy.
Less frequently hypoglossal, trigeminal and accessory nerves.

Morquio's Syndrome

Hereditary disorder affecting ossification of cartilage.
Appears in first two years.
Severe skeletal malformations.
Clouded cornea.

Dwarfism.
Dislocation of hips and genu valgum.
Waddling gait.
Spinal cord compression due to vertebral wedging.
Vascular malformations.
Aortic regurgitation.
Radiological findings include fused cervical vertebrae.
Progresses until growth ceases.
Normal intelligence and life expectancy.

Moschcowitz Syndrome
(Thrombotic Thrombocytopenic Purpura.)

Young adults.
Fibrin and entrapped platelets occlude arterioles in multiple organs.
Haemolytic anaemia.
Thrombocytopenia.
Fever.
Neurological signs.
Renal failure.
Acute course with high mortality.

Munchausen Syndrome

Feign disease in seeking hospital admission.
Usually men.
Onset in twenties.
Tend to avoid psychiatrists.

Munchausen Syndrome By Proxy

Bizarre form of child abuse.
Fictitious illness inflicted on children by their parents.
May result in their being investigated unnecessarily.

Naffziger Syndrome
(v. Cervical Rib Syndrome.)

Nail-Patella Syndrome I

Chromosome 9 disorder.
Absence of patella.
Deformed finger nails.
Dislocated radial heads.
Bilateral iliac bone spurs.

NAME Syndrome

N - naevi.
A - atrial myxoma.
M - mucocutaneous myxomata.
E - ephelids.

Nelson's Syndrome

Follows bilateral adrenalectomy for Cushing's disease.
Marked skin pigmentation.
Pituitary tumour.
Locally invasive.
Enlargement of pituitary fossa.
Pressure on optic chiasma.

Marked skin pigmentation.
May follow bilateral adrenalectomy for Cushing's disease.

Nephrotic Syndrome
(Nephrosis. Epstein Syndrome.)

Severe proteinuria.
Hypoproteinaemic oedema.
Multiple aetiology.
May require renal biopsy for diagnosis.
Glomerulonephritis is commonest cause.
May follow streptococcal ifnection, renal vein thrombosis, lupus erythematosus, diabetes or amyloid disease.

Nezelhof's Syndrome

Variant of severe combined immunodeficiency.
Predominantly T-cell defects.
Deficient immunoglobulin production.
Reduced lymphocyte response.
Impaired immunity predisposes to opportunist infections e.g. candidiasis.

Noonan's Syndrome

Congenital heart disease.
Usually pulmonary valve dysplasia.
Raised right ventricular pressure.
Web neck.
Sternal deformities.
Hypertelorism.
Cryptorchidism in males.
Cafe au lait skin pigmentation.

Ogilvie's Syndrome
(Colonic Pseudo-obstruction.)

Acute dilatation caecum and proximal colon.
Usually stops at splenic flexure.
Considered localised paralytic ileus.
May occur in patients admitted for unconnected major disease
 - myocardial infarct or severe trauma.
Also patients on therapy with neurotoxic drugs, e.g. vincristine.
Caecal perforation can occur but is unusual.
May be recurrent.

Oldfield's Syndrome

Multiple colonic adenomatous polyps.
Multiple sebaceous cysts.

One and a Half Syndrome

Indicates a lesion in the parapontine region.
Failure of lateral conjugate gaze to the same side.
Impaired adduction in eye on that side.
Nystagmus in abduction in opposite eye.
Vertical movements are normal.

Ortner's Syndrome

Mitral stenosis.
Left vocal cord palsy due to enlarged left atrium.

Osler-Rendu-Weber Syndrome
(Hereditary Haemorrhagic Telangiectasis.)

Mendelian dominant vascular disorder.
Spider like or nodular skin telangiectases.
Appear early adult life.
Face, mouth, nose, nail folds.
Mucous membranes.
Rarely pulmonary.

Othello Syndrome

Morbid jealousy.
Accounts for 10% of murders.
Paranoid delusional belief in wife's infidelity.

Pacemaker Syndrome

Retrograde atrio-ventricular conduction causing atrial contractions against closed a-v valves.
Fall in cardiac output and blood pressure.

Page Syndrome

Episodic hypertension, tachycardia, sweating and glycosuria.
Phaeochromocytoma or catecholamine secreting neuroblastoma.

Paget-Schroetter Syndrome

Axillary vein thrombosis.
Aetiology unknown.

Paraneoplastic Syndrome

May present in varying forms.
Signs of ectopic ACTH production in small cell carcinoma of bronchus.
Signs of parathyroid hormone production in squamous cell carcinoma of bronchus.
Peripheral mixed motor-sensory neuropathies.
Signs simulating motor neurone disease.
Signs of cerebellar disease.
Progressive weakness of proximal muscles.
Finger clubbing.
Myasthenia.

Parinaud's Syndrome

Paralysis of voluntary and reflex eye movements.
Eyes will not move up or down vertically.
May or may not have paralysis of convergence.
Lesion in region of aqueduct.

Parkes-Weber Syndrome

Congenital multiple arterio-venous fistulae in a limb.
Pulsatile swelling.
Venous distension.
"Machinery" bruit.
Bony overgrowth with increased length.
Cardiovascular complications leading to heart failure.
Tachycardia falls to normal if main limb artery is compressed (Branham's sign).

Patau's Syndrome
(Trisomy 13.)

Congenital disorder due to extra chromosome 13.
Severe mental retardation.
Microcephaly (small head).
Low set, malformed ears.
Cleft palate and hare lip.
Microphthalmia (small eyes) with colobomata of iris.
Polydactyly (extra digits).
Rocker bottom feet.
Congenital heart disease.
Multiple internal organ malformations.
Most die in first few months.
Commoner in infants born to mothers over 35.

Paterson-Brown-Kelly Syndrome

Hypochromic anaemia.
Dysphagia due to post cricoid web or stricture.
Thought now that anaemia is secondary to the dysphagia rather than the cause of it.

Pellegrini-Stieda Syndrome

Subperiosteal calcification when medial ligament of the knee is torn from its femoral attachment.
Visible on X-Ray as distinct from the adductor tubercle.
Pain on full extension and lateral rotation.

Pendred's Syndrome

Hereditary defect of iodine metabolism.
Iodine does not bond to tyrosine.
Hypothyroidism if defect complete.
Low scrum thyroxin with continued TSH secretion.
Goitre.
Congenital deafness.

Pepper's Syndrome

Abdominal distension.
Caused by extensive liver metastases from neuroblastoma.
Primary usually right adrenal.

Periodic Syndrome

Periodic attacks of various forms for which there is no obvious physical cause.
Often intelligent children of perfectionist parents.
Best known form is "cyclical vomiting".
Vomiting may be severe, lasting 12 to 72 hours.
Often preceded by identifiable trigger.
Often extremely well and vigorous after attack.
May be simply periodic attacks of abdominal pain.

Peutz-Jeghers Syndrome
(Jeghers-Peutz Syndrome.)

Mendelian dominant disorder.
Melanin pigmentation of buccal mucosa.
Mainly lips and inner cheek.

Occasionally face and digits also.
Associated with multiple small bowel adenomata.
Repeated intestinal haemorrhage.

Pfeiffer Syndrome

Autosomal dominant disorder.
Acrocephaly.
Facial dysmorphism.
Stubby thumbs and halluces.
Soft tissue syndactyly.

Pickwickian Syndrome

Complications of extreme obesity.
Dyspnoea and cyanosis due to elevated diaphragm.
Drowsiness and sleep apnoea.
Hypertension and tachycardia.
Polycythaemia.
Cardiac failure.

Pierre-Robin Syndrome

Underdeveloped lower jaw (shrew face).
Tongue falls backwards and downwards (glossoptosis).
Breathing problems at birth.
Cleft palate.
Feeding difficulties.
May occur as part of other syndromes.

Plummer-Vinson Syndrome
(Sideropenic Dysphagia.)

Intermittent dysphagia.

Iron deficiency anaemia.
Glossitis and mucosal atrophy from mouth to stomach.
Koilonychia.
Splenomegaly.
Post cricoid web of atrophic mucosa.

Poland's Syndrome

Unilateral absence of pectoral muscles.
Hypoplastic ribs failing to reach sternum.
Displaced hypoplastic nipple.
Ipsilateral syndactyly.

Posner-Schlossman Syndrome
(Glaucomatocyclitic Crisis.)

Young adults.
Complain of haloes around lights.
Recurrent attacks of glaucoma and uveitis.
Very high pressures for hours or days.
Usually unilateral.

Post Cholecystectomy Syndrome

Post cholecystectomy symptoms for which no cause can be found.
Considered to be biliary tree dysfunction (biliary dyskinesia).
Considerable doubt that condition exists.

Post Concussional Syndrome

Headache.
Vertigo.
Memory loss.

Lack of concentration.
Depression and anxiety.
No obvious organic basis.

Post Hepatitis Syndrome

Prolonged debility after clinical recovery from acute Type A hepatitis.
Malaise, anorexia and nausea.
No clinical or biochemical abnormality to be found.

Post Myocardial Infarct Syndrome
(Dressler's Syndrome.)

Fever, pericarditis and pleurisy.
Weeks or months after infarct.
Autoimmune reaction to dead myocardium.
Often subsides after few days.

Postphlebitic Syndrome

Follows occlusion of major veins, usually lower limb.
Persistent swelling.
Aggravated by standing.
Feeling of heaviness.
Varicosities form in collateral superficial veins.
Eczema.
Indolent, gravitational ulceration.

Potter Syndrome

Oligohydramnos and foetal compression due to renal agenesis.

Epicanthic folds.
Flattened nose and low set ears.
Receding chin.
Urogenital malformations.
Leg deformities.
Survival depends largely on degree of pulmonary hypoplasia also present.

Prader-Labhart-Willi Syndrome

Obesity due to increased appetite.
Appetite thought to be induced by release of endogenous endorphins.
Appetite inhibited by narcotic antagonists.
Dwarfism.
Marked hypotonia.
Mental retardation.
Hypogonadism and cryptorchidism.
May develop diabetes mellitus.

Prune Belly Syndrome
(Eagle-Barrett Syndrome.)

Almost exclusively male children.
Deficient abdominal muscles.
Slack, wrinkled abdominal wall.
Genitourinary malformations including patent urachus.
Bilateral undescended testes.
Pulmonary hypoplasia may be fatal.

Raeder's Syndrome

Damage to sympathetic plexus in carotid sheat.
Horner's syndrome mnus facial anhidrosis.
Associated with lesion of 1st division of the trigeminal nerve.
Loss of corneal sensation often earliest feature.
Caused by lesion at the base of the skull.

Ramsay-Hunt Syndrome
(Geniculate Herpes Zoster.)

Shingles in distribution of trigeminal nerve.
Infranuclear facial paresis.
Hyperacusis.
Unilateral loss of taste.
Vertigo.

Ramsay-Hunt Syndrome
(Dyssynergia Cerebellaris Myoclonica.)

Disease of childhood.
Sudden myoclonic jerking.
Mild progressive cerebellar ataxia.
Mild seizure disorder.
Many metabolic and degenerative causes.

Rapunzel Syndrome

Large trichobezoar extending from stomach throughout small intestine.
Weight loss.
Anaemia.
Intestinal obstruction.

Refsum's Syndrome

Intracellular enzyme disorder (lysosomal disease).
Neurological complications at birth or early childhood.
Earliest symptom often night blindness.
Peripheral neuropathy.
Cerebellar incoordination.
Retinitis pigmentosa.
Dry, scaly skin rash.

Respiratory Distress Syndrome
(RDS. Hyaline Membrane Disease.)

Hyaline membrane may be result rather than cause.
Particularly premature newborns.
Commonest cause of death in preterm infants.
Rarely affects mature infants.
Predisposing factors antepartum haemorrhage, diabetes mellitus.
Caused by substance (surfactant) which prevents alveolar collapse during expiration.
Breathing difficulties.
Cyanosis.
Arterial hypoxaemia.

Restless Legs Syndrome
(Ekbom Syndrome.)

Troublesome restlessness disturbing rest.
Leg cramps.
Often occurs in elderly with diabetes, uraemia, cerebrovascular disease, drug therapy.

Rett Syndrome
(Cerebroatrophic Hyperammonaemia.)

Progressive neurological disorder.
Female children only.
Onset about one year.
Development ceases after 9th to18th month.
Failure of head to grow.
Epilepsy.
Mental retardation.
Autism.
Ataxia.
Compulsive hand movements.

Reye's Syndrome

Acute neurological disorder of mitochondrial function in brain and liver.
Complication of viral infection.
Up to 18 years but usually very young children.
Nausea and vomiting.
Lethargy and drowsiness.
Cerebral oedema.
Confusion with disorientation leading to coma.
Abnormal liver function tests.
Hypoglycaemia.
May develop pancreatitis.
Respiratory arrest.
May follow aspirin, aflatoxin or warfarin therapy.

Richardson-Steele-Olszewski Syndrome
(Progressive Supranuclear Palsy.)

Gait disturbance and falls.
Memory loss.
Personality change due to subcortical dementia.
Failure of voluntary eye movement, particularly downward gaze.
Axial rigidity with extended postures.
May mimic Parkinson's disease in early stages.

Riddoch Syndrome

Defect of vision in one lateral half of visual field.
Recognise objects only when attention is drawn to them.
Lesion between thalamus and occipital lobe.

Rieger's Syndrome

Reduced number of teeth.
Abnormally small teeth.
Maxillary hypoplasia.
Hypertelorism.
Iris defects (Rieger's anomaly).

Riley-Day Syndrome
(Dysautonomia.)

Almost exclusively in Jews.
Emotional instability.
Postural hypotension.
Dysphagia due to incoordination.
Sweating and skin changes when eating or excited.

Crying without tears.
Relative indifference to pain.

Robin Hood Syndrome
(Inverse Steal Syndrome.)

Blood flow to cerebral damage is above metabolic needs (v. luxury perfusion syndrome).
Reducing carbon dioxide levels induces vasoconstriction in normal cerebral tissue.
Perfusion of damaged cerebral tissue thereby increased even further.

Rothmund's Syndrome
(Rothmund-Thomson Syndrome.)

Hereditary.
Predominantly females.
Early infancy.
Skin changes - marble skin, pigmentation, telangiectasis.
Bony defects.
Hypogonadism.
Cataracts from ten years onwards (may be congenital).

Rotor Syndrome

Rare disorder of bilirubin storage in liver cells.
Mild jaundice.
Hyperbilirubinaemia (conjugated).
Bile in urine.
Normal liver histology.
Prognosis excellent.

Roussy-Levy Syndrome
(v. Levy-Roussy Syndrome.)

Rubinstein-Taybi Syndrome

Mental and physical retardation.
Microcephaly.
Eyes wide apart.
Ptosis and squints.
High arched palate.
Broad, flat big toes and thumbs.
Undescended testes.
Cardiac and renal malformations.

Russell-Silver Syndrome
(Silver Syndrome.)

Slender short stature.
Asymmetry of limbs with large skull.
Premature sexual maturity.
Wide forehead and narrow chin giving triangular facial appearance.
Inturned little fingers.
Cafe-au-lait spots on body.
Relatively favourable prognosis.

Russell Syndrome
(Diencephalic Syndrome.)

Weight loss.
Tremor.
Ataxia.
Nystagmus.

Euphoria.
Diencephalic tumour.

Sandifer's Syndrome

Spasmodic contortions of face and head.
Similar to torticollis.
Found occasionally with gastro-oesophageal reflux.

Sanfillipo's Syndrome

Rare recessive, hereditary disorder of mucopolysaccharide metabolism.
Appears in early childhood.
Hirsutism.
Degree of dwarfism.
Severe mental deficiency.
May be hyperactivity with destructive behaviour.
Progressive partial paralysis of all four limbs.
Rarely survive beyond 20 years.

Scalded Skin Syndrome
(Lyell's Disease. Ritter's Disease.)

Epidermal necrolysis due to toxins of staphylococcus type 71.
Acute skin infection develops into generalised skin exfoliation.
May also follow certain therapeutic drugs.
Slightest trauma results in loss of skin.

Scalenus Anticus Syndrome
(v. Cervical Rib Syndrome.)

Scheie's Syndrome
(Variant of Hurler's Syndrome)

Rare hereditary disorder of mucopolysaccharide metabolism.
Corneal clouding.
Claw hands.
Aortic incompetence.
Carpal tunnel syndrome.
Differs from Hurler's syndrome in that -
  No dwarfism.
  Normal intelligence and life span.

Shakhonovich's Syndrome
(Hypokalaemic Periodic Paralysis.)

Autosomal dominant.
Usually presents 7 - 21 years.
Flaccid paralysis beginning in the legs.
Spreads rest of body.
Typically starts early morning.
Precipitated by various factors - stress, menstruation, cold, large carbohydrate meal.
Recovery takes up to 24 hours.
Very low sodium diet may prevent attacks.

Sheehan's Syndrome
(Postpartum Pituitary Necrosis.)

Anterior pituitary disorder causing hypopituitarism.
Infarction may follow hypotension from haemorrhage, burns or severe sepsis.
Commonest after pregnancy.
Failure to lactate.

Symptoms may not appear until several years after the event.
Amenorrhoea.
Skin pallor.
Loss of secondary sexual characteristics.
Loss of body hair.
In male - impotence, loss of libido, gynaecomastia.

Short Gut Syndrome

Follows massive small bowel resection.
Occasionally after jejuno-ileal bypass for gross obesity.
Extensive ileal resection greater effect than jejunal due to inability to absorb bile salts and Vit B12.
Retention of ileocaecal valve beneficial in slowing transit and reducing retrograde colonisation of small bowel.
30 cms of small bowel supports nutrition.
Malabsorption mainly fats and proteins.
Calcium and magnesium precipitate as soaps with unabsorbed fatty acids.

Shoulder-Hand Syndrome

Pain in shoulder.
Pain, swelling and stiffness in hand with vasomotor changes.
Cervical spondylitis may be found.
May follow myocardial infarction, breast or thoracic surgery.
May be idiopathic.
Tend to occur in hysterical personalities.

Shy-Drager Syndrome

Progressive autonomic failure.

Primary orthostatic hypotension.
No cardiac response to posture or exercise.
Sweating disorder (anhidrosis).
Horner's syndrome.
Cricopharyngeal crises.
Bowel function disorder.
Impotence.
Severe sleep apnoea.

Sicca Syndrome

Dryness of eyes, mouth (xerostoma), respiratory passages.
Salivary gland enlargement and malignancy.
Dysphagia.
Dyspareunia.
Dental caries.
Hepatosplenomegaly.
Raynaud's phenomenon.
Thyroiditis.
Pancreatitis.
Purpura.
Pulmonary fibrosis.
Long term - reticulum cell sarcoma and primary macroglobulinaemia.

Sick Sinus Syndrome

Any age, commonly elderly.
Bradycardia and syncope.
Sinus arrest (absent P waves on ECG).
Paroxysmal tachycardia.
Best diagnosed with ambulatory continuous ECG.

Silver Syndrome
(v. Russell-Silver Syndrome.)

Sipple's Syndrome
(Multiple Endocrine Neoplasia. MEN 2.)

Thyroid medullary carcinoma.
Phaeochromocytoma.
Multiple neuromata.
Hyperparathyroidism.
Marfan-like characteristics.
Cushing's syndrome (rare).

Sjogren's Syndrome

Mostly postmenopausal women.
Dryness of eyes, mouth (xerostoma), respiratory passages.
Over half develop rheumatoid arthritis.
Raynaud's phenomenon.
Thyroiditis.
Less commonly associated with scleroderma, polymyositis, systemic lupus erythematosus, polyarteritis nodosa, myasthenia gravis.
Non-Hodgkin's lymphoma.

Sjorgen-Larsson Syndrome

Very rare autosomal recessive disorder.
Both sexes.
Icthyosis (fish scale skin).
Spasticity particularly of lower limbs.
Mental handicap.
Retinal degeneration.

Sly Syndrome

Variant of Hurler's syndrome.

Smith-Lemli-Opitz Syndrome

Autosomal recessive.
Microcephaly.
Congenital ptosis.
Simian creases.
Cryptorchidism.
Hypospadias.
Severe mental deficiency.

Sotos Syndrome
(Cerebral Gigantism.)

Hereditary but sporadic amongst a family.
May also follow pre- or perinatal hypoxic damage to hypothalamus.
Early rapid growth through first 4 to 5 years.
Bone age and tooth eruption are advanced.
Macrocephaly and prominent forehead.
Eyes wide apart.
Large chin.
High arched palate.
Clumsy large limbs.
Mild mental retardation.
Renal tumours, particularly Wilm's.

Stauffer's Syndrome

Hepato-splenomegaly.
Raised alkaline phosphatase.
Hypernephroma (Grawitz tumour).

Steak House Syndrome

Sudden obstruction by food bolus at lower end oesophagus.
Usually associated with previously symptomless Schatzki's ring.

Steal Syndrome

Obstruction origin of left subclavian artery.
Pressure beyond the obstruction is lowered.
Blood syphons retrogradely down left vertebral artery.
Results in cerebral ischaemia.

Stein-Leventhal Syndrome

Endocrine disorder in women due to increased androgen secretion.
Becomes apparent at puberty.
Mild degrees may go undiagnosed.
Anovulation.
Irregular menses or amenorrhoea.
Infertility.
Obesity, hirsutism and acne.
Polycystic ovaries.

Stevens-Johnson Syndrome

Severe erythema multiforme of skin and conjunctivae.
Mucous membrane ulceration.

Adverse effect of sulphonamide therapy.
May be fatal.

Stickler Syndrome
(Arthro-Ophthalmopathy.)

Autosomal dominant.
Flat, asymmetrical face.
Cleft palate.
Myopia.
Glaucoma, cataract, retinal detachment leading to blindness.
Hypotonic musculature.
Lax joints.
Mild to severe rheumatoid arthropathy.

Stiffman's Syndrome
(Myositis Ossificans.)

Muscle replaced by bone.
May be localised (myositis ossificans circumscripta).
May follow trauma.
May be progressive (myositis ossificans progressiva).
Extends from one muscle group to another.
Difficulty in breathing.
Dysphagia.
Death from respiratory infection.

Stokes-Adams Syndrome

Cardiac syncope.
May occur without warning.
Convulsions if asystole prolonged.
Pallor with characteristic flush on recovery.

Usually intermittent heart block.
Failure of escape mechanism in chronic, complete heart block.
Sick sinus syndrome.

Stuart-Treves Syndrome

Multiple angiosarcomata in the skin of the arm.
May metastasise to lungs.
Occur in women with long standing, severe lymphoedema following radical mastectomy and radiotherapy.

Sturge-Weber Syndrome

Vascular "port wine" skin lesion over upper face and skull.
Distribution first branch trigeminal nerve.
Corresponding intracranial lesions.
Contralateral convulsions.
Spastic hemiparesis.
Visual field defects.
Radiology shows "tram line" type of intracranial calcification.
Mental deterioration ultimately develops.

Sudden Infant Death Syndrome
(SIDS. Cot death. Crib death.)

Most common at two weeks to four months.
Commonest cause of death from two weeks to one year.
During sleep.
Cause unknown.
Theories, mostly discarded, include parental neglect, apnoea, poor prenatal care, mothers who smoke, position of infant during sleep.

Supermale Syndrome
(XYY Trisomy.)

Chromosomal disorder.
Males have extra Y chromosome.
Tall.
Severe acne.
Mental retardation.
May be connected with abnormally aggressive behaviour.

Taravana Syndrome
(v. Caisson disease.)

Decompression sickness in pearl divers.
Joint pains.
Paralysis.

Tarsal Tunnel Syndrome

Compression of posterior tibial nerve beneath fibrous arch from which abductor hallucis takes its origin.
Pain, numbness and paraesthesiae in distribution of posterior tibial nerve.
Predisposing factors include anything likely to cause oedema, myxoedema, diabetes mellitus and rheumatoid arthritis.

Tietze's Syndrome

M : F :: 1 : 2
Tender, swollen costochondral junction.
Usually left sided.
One cause of chest pain.
May mimic breast pain.

Tolosa Hunt Syndrome

IIIrd, IVth and VIth nerve palsies giving painful ophthalmoplegia.
Caused by granulomatous vasculitis of carotid artery.
Raised ESR.

Tourette's Syndrome
(Gilles de la Tourette's Syndrome.)

Rare, usually inherited.
M : F :: 3 : 1
Onset usually 2 to 15 years.
Neurological basis rather than psychiatric.
Motor tics, often facial, may be more complex.
Motor tic often preceded by vocal tic interrupting normal speech.
Also heard may be -
    Coprolalia - obscene utterings.
    Echolalia - repetition of words spoken by others.
    Palilalia - repetition of own words.

Toxic Shock Syndrome

Caused by toxaemia from certain strains of staphylococcus aureus.
Usually in women using types of tampons.
High fever.
Headache.
Vomiting.
Irritability.
Severe hypotension.
Respiratory distress.
Renal failure.

Treacher-Collins Syndrome
(Francheschetti-Klein Syndrome.
Mandibulofacial Dysostosis.)

Rare, dominant hereditary genetic disorder.
Underdeveloped facial bones and lower jaw.
Hypertelorism.
Malformation of lower eyelid.
No eyelashes.
No external auditory canal.
Deafness.
Normal intelligence.

Turcot's Syndrome

Colonic adenomata with central nervous system tumours.
Medulloblastoma.
Ependymoma.
Astrocytoma.

Turner's Syndrome

Sex chromosome disorder in females.
Not related to mother's age.
Low hairline.
Webbed neck.
Broad chest with widely spaced nipples.
Cubitus valgus (increased carrying angle at elbow).
Heart malformation often with coarctation of aorta.
Low I.Q. with 10% mentally retarded.
Absent ovaries and amenorrhoea.
Failure to develop at puberty.
May develop a male body type.

Urethral Syndrome

Symptoms of cystitis or urethritis with a sterile urine.
Predominantly female.
Cause unknown.

Usher's Syndrome

Autosomal recessive disorder.
Both sexes.
90% born with profound deafness.
Retinitis pigmentosa.
Visual defects beginning about 10 years with loss of peripheral vision.
Glaucoma and cataracts.
Progression to total blindness.
Ataxia.

van Buchem Syndrome

Thickening base of skull and mandible.
Raised alkaline phosphatase.
Stenosis exit foramina of skull.
Optic atrophy.
Deafness.
Facial palsy.

van der Hoeve Syndrome
(Osteogenesis Imperfecta Tarda.)

Hereditary.
Normal at birth (c.f. osteogenesis imperfecta congenita).
Multiple fractures during childhood.
Incidence of fractures reduces after puberty.

Blue sclera.
Deafness.
Double jointed.
Thin skinned.

Verner-Morrison Syndrome
(Pancreatic Cholera. WDHA Syndrome.)

Watery diarrhoea.
Hypokalaemia (and acidosis).
Achlorhydria.
Islet cell tumour usual cause.
50% tumours malignant.
Secrete vasoactive intestinal polypeptide (VIP) (vipoma).
Lethargy and weakness.
Colic and weight loss.
Also described with oat cell tumour of lung, malignant carcinoids, medullary carcinomas of thyroid, ganglioneuromata and neuroblastomas.

Vernet's Syndrome

Damage to three nerves that traverse the jugular foramen, i.e. IXth, Xth and XIth.
Usually due to intracranial lesion (cf. Collet-Sicard syndrome).

Villaret's Syndrome

Damage to last four cranial nerves together with Horner's syndrome.
Due to lesion in retropharyngeal space.

Vogt-Koyanagi-Harada Syndrome

Alopecia.
Poliosis.
Vitiligo.
Headaches with meningism.
Cranial nerve palsies and convulsions.
Tinnitus, vertigo and deafness.
CSF high lymphocyte count.
Iridocyclitis.
Retinal detachment (Harada).

Waardenburg's Syndrome

Autosomal dominant disorder.
Probably chromosome 9.
Both sexes.
Widely separated eyes with confluent eyebrows.
Eyes different colour, e.g. one blue, one brown.
Glaucoma.
Small nose.
White forelock.
Sensori-neural deafness.
May have varying degree of upper limbs' failure to develop.

Wallenberg Syndrome

Posterior inferior cerebellar artery thrombosis.
Ipsilateral hemiataxia and hemianaesthesia.
Contralateral loss of pain and temperature sensation.
Ipsilateral paralysis of larynx and palate.

Waterhouse-Friderichsen Syndrome

Occurs in septiceamia.
Usually meningococcal but may be streptococcal or pneumococcal.
High fever with possible coma.
Haemorrhage into skin and mucosae.
Severe collapse due to haemorrhage into adrenal cortex.
Death may occur within hours, before overt signs of meningitis appear.

Weaver Syndrome

Form of childhood gigantism.
Congenital macrosomia.
Macrocephaly.
Increased muscle tone.
Deep hoarse voice.
Psychomotor retardation.

Weber's Syndrome

Lesion in pyramidal tracts in region of the crus with simultaneous involvement of IIIrd cranial nerve.
Contralateral upper motor neurone paralysis of face, arm and leg.
Ipsilateral lower motor neurone ophthalmoplegia and ptosis.

Weill-Marchesani Syndrome
(Dystrophia Mesodermalis Hyperplasia.)

Short stature.
Short stubby fingers (brachydactyly).
Mental retardation.
Spherophakia.

Myopia and glaucoma.
Ocular lens dislocation.

Wermer's Syndrome
(Multiple Endocrine Neoplasia. MEN 1.)

Autosomal dominant.
Hyperparathyroidism.
Pancreatic tumours (gastrinoma; insulinoma).
Hyperinsulinism.
Anterior pituitary hyperplasia (acidophil or chromophobe adenomata).
Adrenal hyperplasia and carcinoid tumours (rare).
Thyroid tumours (rare).
Zollinger-Ellison and Verner-Morrison syndromes may coexist.

Werner's Syndrome
(Adult Progeria.)

Recessive hereditary trait.
Premature ageing appearing in young adulthood or adolescence.
Develop physical attributes of old age.
Susceptible to diseases of old age.
CNS is exempt.
No senility.
Appear about 30 years older than they are.
No dwarfism.
Sexually mature but underdeveloped external genitalia.
Balding, loss of teeth, deafness, cataracts, osteoporosis, heart disease.
Average life span is 47 years.

Wernicke-Korsakoff Syndrome

Vitamin B deficiency, common in alcoholics.
Cerebellar incoordination.
Ocular palsies.
Nystagmus.
Mental confusion with amnesia.
Confabulation - fabrication of memories compensating true memory loss.
Peripheral neuropathy.

West's Syndrome
(Hypsarrhythmia.)

Failure of normal cerebral activity.
Probably metabolic disorder (phenyl-ketonuria).
May follow period of anoxia at birth.
Fits, beginning from birth to 2 years.
Rapid succession of jerks into flexed position before returning to normal.
May involve head only.
Cerebral anomalies usually found on CAT scan.
10% will develop normally.
Remainder mentally handicapped.
May develop other features of epilepsy.

Williams Syndrome
(Infantile Hypercalcaemia.)

Autosomal disorder of calcium metabolism.
Both sexes.
Round, chubby faces.

Physical retardation.
Hyperactive by day, sleepless by night.
Behavioural problems.
Heart defects, particularly aortic stenosis.
Hyperacute hearing.
Renal calculi.

Wiskott-Aldrich Syndrome
(Familial Thrombocytopenia.)

Thrombocytopenia due to hereditary cellular immunodeficiency disorder.
Sex linked - males only.
Severe thrombocytopenia.
Eczema.
Repeated infections with various micro-organisms.
Asthma.
Purpura.
Most children die from overwhelming infection.
Others die from lymphoma or leukaemia.

Wolff-Parkinson-White Syndrome

Paroxysmal tachycardia.
Due to band of conducting tissue bypassing AV node.
Bypass conducts faster than via AV node.
Normal QRS complexes during tachycardia.
At risk of ventricular tachycardia, ventricular fibrillation and death if auricle is fibrillating as AV rate limitation ability is also bypassed.

Wolf-Hirschorn Syndrome
(Wolf's Syndrome.)

Congenital chromosome 4 disorder.
Hypertelorism.
Prominent glabella.
Beaked nose.
Cleft lip and palate.
Micrognathia.
Genital malformations.

Young's Syndrome

Recurrent chest infections.
Sinusitis.
Epididymal obstruction.
Infertility.

Zellweger Syndrome
(Cerebro-Hepato-Renal Syndrome.)

Autosomal recessive metabolic dysplasia.
Extreme muscular hypotonia.
Absent deep tendon reflexes.
Hepatomegaly.
Absent psychomotor development.
Deafness.
Early death.

Zollinger-Ellison Syndrome

Non-beta-cell pancreatic tumour (gastrinoma) or hyperplasia of pancreatic islets.

Excessive gastrin secretion.
Gastric parietal cell stimulation produces hyperacidity.
Severe multiple gastric ulceration.
Jejunal and oesophageal ulceration may also occur.
Upper small bowel pH reduced, inactivating pancreatic lipase.
Diarrhoea and steatorrhoea.
May present as recurrent gastro-intestinal ulceration after gastric surgery.
High levels of circulating gastrin.
25% have MEN 1 syndrome with no peripancreatic tumour.

Zuelzer-Wilson Syndrome

Variant of Hirschsprung's disease.
Aganglionic segment not restricted to rectosigmoid.
May be total throughout large bowel.

Signs

Adie Pupil
(Holmes-Adie Pupil.)
Probably Partial Parasympathetic Denervation

Young healthy adults.
More frequently females.
Absent or delayed constriction both to light and accommodation.
Impaired parasympathetic supply to pupillary muscle.
80% unilateral, giving unequal pupils (anisocoria).
Pupil tonically dilated but may be found constricted.
Dilates slowly in the dark.
Constriction to light or accommodation is slow.
Varies in size but never reacts promptly.
Constricts with instillation of 2% methacholine, c.f. Argyll Robertson pupil which does not.
Diminished tendon reflexes.
Impaired sweating.
Usually of no clinical importance.

Adson Test
Thoracic Outlet Compression

Raise chin.
Rotate head.
Radial pulse disappears.

Alder's Sign
Genital Tract Disease

Palpate abdomen lying flat.
Locate site of pain.
Turn patient on left side with hand still in place.

If pain shifts to the left, likely to arise in uterus or adnexae.
If pain does not shift, likely to be extragenital in origin.

Allen Test
Vascular Supply to Hand

Raise arm.
Make a tight fist.
Compress radial artery.
Lower arm.
Persistent pallor of hand denotes deficient ulnar arterial supply.
Repeat with ulnar artery compression.

Allis Sign (Galleazi Sign)
Congenital Dislocation of Hip

Place baby on firm surface.
Flex both hips.
Press buttocks against firm surface.
One hip will appear shorter than the other.

Apley's Test
Knee Joint Trauma

Patient lies prone.
Flex knee to 90°.
Rotate while compressing joint.
Pain suggests torn meniscus.
Examiner places his knee on patient's thigh to hold leg down.
Leg is raised to distract joint.
Pain on rotation suggests ligamental damage.

Argyll Robertson Pupil
Neurosyphilis

Small, irregular, unequal pupils.
Do not react to light but do so on convergence.
Typically bilateral but often more obvious on one side.
Dilates only slowly to atropine.

Aschoff Nodule
Rheumatic Fever

Granuloma found in heart muscle.
Specific to rheumatic fever.

Austin Flint Murmur
Aortic Regurgitation

Low pitched diastolic murmur in mitral area in presence of severe aortic regurgitation.
May resemble murmur of mitral stenosis but mitral cusps are normal.
No opening snap.

Babinski "Rising Up" Sign
Spastic Paralysis Lower Limb

Patient lies supine with legs extended.
Required to raise up without using his arms.
In spastic paralysis of a leg, the limb will rise first.
In hysterical paralysis, this does not happen.

Babinski's Sign
Pyramidal Tract Lesion

Extensor plantar response with slow dorsiflexion of the great toe and spreading of the small toes.
Dorsiflexion of ankle and flexion of knee may follow.
Pathognomonic of upper motor neurone lesion.
Unreliable in infants.

Bainbridge Reflex
Raised Right Atrial Pressure

Increased heart rate in raised right atrial pressure.

Ballance's Sign
Ruptured Spleen

Dullness in both flanks, shifting on the right, fixed on the left.
Pathognomonic of ruptured spleen.

Barlow's Test
Congenital Dislocation of the Hip

Newborn lies supine.
Flex and adduct both hips.
With finger over greater trochanter, lift hip up into socket, abducting lightly (cf.Ortolani's test).

Battle's Sign
Fracture Posterior Cranial Fossa

Discolouration near tip of the mastoid process due to blood following the track of the posterior auricular artery.

Baumann's Angle
Supracondylar Fracture of Humerus

Radiological angle between capitellum and shaft of humerus.
Important to restore to avoid cubitus varus after reduction.

Beau's Lines
Any Severe Illness

Transverse ridges on finger nails.
May date the onset of any serious illness.

Beck's Triad
Cardiac Tamponade

Low arterial pressure.
High venous pressure.
Absent apex beat.

Bell's Reflex
Thermal Eye Injuries

Eye is protected by reflexly turning upwards as eyelids blink.

Bernstein's Test
Acid Oesophageal Reflux

Infuse the oesophagus first with saline.
Then infuse with acid.
Repeat both phases at least once.
Symptoms of retrosternal pain may correlate with those complained of.

Berry's Sign
Malignant Goitre

Difficulty in palpating the carotid artery.
Unlike in benign goitres, when the carotid sheath is displaced, the artery becomes involved in the tumour.

Bishop's Score
Induction of Labour

Mathematical assessment of chances of success in inducing labour.
Five factors taken into calculation.
- Dilatation of cervix.
- Effacement.
- Station of presenting part.
- Consistency of cervix.
- Position of cervix.

Bitot's Spots
Vitamin A Deficiency

Desquamating, hyperkeratotic conjunctival plaques.
Usually lateral margin of cornea.
Triangular in shape.

Boas Sign
Acute Cholecystitis

Area of epicritic hyperaesthesia posteriorly below right scapula.

Bouchard's Nodes
Osteoarthritis

Similar to Heberden's nodes but occurring on proximal interphalangeal joints.

Branham's Sign
Arterio-venous Fistula

Tachycardia in presence of significant arterio-venous fistula drops to normal rate on compression of main artery to limb involved.

Broadbent Sign
Constrictive Pericarditis

Indrawing of 11th and 12th ribs due to pericardial adhesion to diaphragm.

Brodie-Trendelenberg Percussion Test
Varicose Veins

Test for incompetent valves in superficial veins.
One finger placed on lower end of vein to be examined.
Vein percussed at upper end.
Palpable impulse denotes incompetence.

Brudzinski's Sign
Meningitis

Flexion of the legs when the neck is passively flexed on the chest.
Passive flexion of one thigh results in flexion of opposite hip and knee.

Brushfield Spots
Mongolism

White or yellow pinpoint spots in infant iris in Downs Syndrome

Burton Line
Lead or Copper Poisoning

Dark blue discolouration of gums.
Most obvious with poor oral hygiene.

Cafe-au-lait Spots
Neurofibromatosis

Large pigmented patches.
Also in Albright's syndrome.

Campbell de Morgan Spots
No Clinical Significance

Senile skin haemangiomata.
Thought at one time to indicate some malignancy.

Caput Medusae
Portal Hypertension

Prominent veins around umbilicus from collateral circulation.

Carvallo's Sign
Tricuspid Incompetence

Murmur increased on inspiration.

Charcot's Triad
Multiple Sclerosis

Intention tremor.
Nystagmus.
Slurred speech.
Sign of brain stem involvement.

Chevrier's Percussion Test
Varicose Veins

Patient stands with veins distended.
Tap lower end of vein.
Percussion wave is felt on light touch over upper end of vein.

Cheyne-Stokes Respiration
Cardiac Failure

Periodic variation in depth of respiration.
Recurring hyperpnoea followed by apnoea.
Ranges from hyperventilation to apnoea lasting perhaps 30 seconds.
Common in cardiac failure, renal failure, increased intracranial pressure and narcotic poisoning.
May also be seen in the elderly.

Chvostek Sign
(Chvostek-Weiss Sign.)
Tetany

Percussion over facial nerve produces spasm of the facial muscles.
10 - 15% normal patients may have positive result.

Codman's Sign
Supraspinatus Tendon Rupture

Passive abduction of the shoulder is painless.
Attempted active abduction is painful.

Codman's Triangle
Osteosarcoma

Radiological sign.
New bone formed under periosteum raised at the margins of a sarcoma.

Corrigan's Pulse
Aortic Incompetence

Collapsing (water hammer) pulse.
Characteristic of free aortic regurgitation.

Courvoisier's Law
Obstructive Jaundice

If, in a case of obstructive jaundice, the gall bladder is palpable, the cause of the jaundice is likely to be something other than gall stones.

Cruveilhier's Sign
Saphenous Varix

Palpable thrill, likened to a jet of water, over varix on coughing.

Cullen's Sign
Ruptured Ectopic Pregnancy

Bluish discolouration around umbilicus.
May also occur in pancreatitis.

Cushing Reflex
Raised Intracranial Pressure

Slow pulse.
Raised blood pressure.
Result of sudden rise in intracranial pressure.

Dalrymple's Sign
Thyrotoxicosis

Widened palpebral fissure due to upper lid spasm.

Darier's Sign
Urticaria

Stroking the skin produces erythema and oedema.

Drawer Test
Knee Joint Instability

Flex knee to 90°.
Rock tibia backwards and forwards.
Test for cruciate laxity.
Excessive anterior movement - lax anterior cruciate ligament.
Excessive posterior movement - lax posterior cruciate ligament.

Dugas's Sign
Dislocated Shoulder

Place hand of affected side on opposite shoulder.
Elbow cannot touch the chest wall.

Fawn's Tail
Spina Bifida Occulta

Abnormally heavy growth hair on lower back.
Suggests underlying neural malformation.

Finkelstein's Test
de Quervain's Stenosing Tenosynovitis

Pain on abducting thumb against resistance.
Pain on passive adduction of thumb across the palm.

Froment's Sign
Ulnar Palsy

Paralysis of adductor pollicis.
Thumb flexes when holding paper between thumb and forefinger.

Galleazzi Sign (Allis Sign)
Congenital Dislocation of Hip

Place baby on firm surface.
Flex both hips.
Press buttocks against firm surface.
One hip will appear shorter than the other.

Goodsall's Rule
Anal Fistula

Draw a line horizontally across anus.
All fistulae with external openings posterior to the line open internally in the midline.
All fistulae with external openings anterior to this line have internal openings at corresponding radial point.

Gordon's Sign
Pyramidal Tract Lesion

Extensor response, similar to Babinski, on squeezing the calf muscles.

Gower Sign
Duchenne Muscular Dystrophy

Child uses his hands and arms to "climb up himself" to assume the vertical position.

Graham Steel Murmur
Pulmonary Hypertension

Pulmonary early diastolic murmur due to pulmonary regurgitation. Heard best at left sternal edge.

Grey Turner's Sign
Haemorrhagic Pancreatitis

Discolouration in both flanks.
Normally first seen on left side

Gunn's Pupil
Optic nerve Lesion

Test of consensual reaction to light.
Shine light in one eye.
Switch light suddenly to other eye.
Initial contraction may be followed by dilatation (pupillary escape phenomenon).
Dilatation rather than constriction suggests consensual reaction is stronger than direct.
Indicates a lesion in the optic nerve.
Useful sign in retrobulbar neuritis.
Also compression or ischaemia of optic nerve.

Hamman's Sign
Mediastinal Emphysema

Clicking or crunching sound ("clicking pneumothorax").
Synchronous with heart beat.
Air in mediastinum.
Ruptured bronchus.
After thoracotomy.

Harrison's Sulci
Congenital Heart Disease. Asthma.
Chronic Respiratory Infection. Infantile Rickets

Depressions in chest wall.
Run parallel to but above the diaphragmatic attachment.
Often associated with unduly prominent sternum.

Heberden's Nodes
Osteoarthritis

Bony nodules base of terminal phalanges.
Indicates osteoarthritis small joints.

Hess Test
Bleeding Disorders

Test of capillary resistance.
Inflate blood pressure cuff to 80 mm Hg.
Determine number of petechiae in antecubital fossa.
Not specific for bleeding disorders.
May appear in health, infectious diseases and chronic renal disease.
Not always positive in thrombocytopenia.

Hilgenreiner's Line
Congenital Dislocation of Hip

Horizontal radiological line drawn between both acetabular triradiate cartilages (v. Perkin's line).
Femoral head should lie below this line.

Hochsinger's Sign
Tetany

Closure of the fist on compression of the biceps muscle.
Sign of hypocalcaemia.

Homan's Sign
Deep Vein Thrombosis

Forceful dorsiflexion of the foot causes pain, tightness and tenderness in the calf.

Horsley's Sign
Middle Meningeal Haemorrhage

Temperatures taken in both axillae may show a degree difference. Raised on the paralysed side.

Howship-Romberg Sign
Obturator Nerve Compression

Pain and paraesthesiae down inner side of thigh as far as knee.
Made worse by extending hip with either internal rotation or adduction.
Any cause of obturator nerve compression.
Most commonly obturator hernia.

Hutchinson's Sign
Herpes Zoster

Lesions side of nose due to nasociliary nerve involvement.
Correlates closely with subsequent ocular complications.

Hutchinson's Sign
Middle Meningeal Haemorrhage

Initial contraction of pupil on side of compression, followed by gradual dilatation and loss of light sensitivity.

Hutchinson's Teeth
Congenital Syphilis

Rounded, peg shaped, notched upper incisors. Now rare.

Hutchinson's Triad
Congenital Syphilis

Deafness.
Interstitial keratitis.
Pointed teeth.

Jendrassik's Manoeuvre
Parkinsonism

Cogwheel rigidity of extrapyramidal origin is enhanced by simultaneous contraction of another muscle, e.g. by making a fist.

Joffroy's Sign
Exophthalmos

Absence of forehead wrinkling on looking upwards.

Kanavel's Sign
Ulnar bursitis

Maximal tenderness in palm over hypothenar eminence.

Kantor String Sign
Crohn's Disease

Radiological sign.
Long narrow stricture in terminal ileum.

Kehr's Sign
Ruptured Spleen

Hyperaesthesia over left shoulder.
Subdiaphragmatic irritation in haemoperitoneum.

Kenawy's Sign
Hepatosplenomegaly

Audible hum on auscultation over liver, louder on inspiration.
Thought to be due to splenic vein engorgement.

Kernig's Sign
Bacterial Meningitis

Flex the thigh to 90° to the abdomen.
The knee cannot then be straightened passively as stretching sciatic nerve roots, inflamed in the spinal theca, causes spasm of the hamstrings.

Kestenbaum's Sign
Optic Atrophy

Reduction of number of capillaries crossing the disc margin to 7 or less.

Kocher's Sign
Thyrotoxicosis

Wide eyed frightened stare.

Koplik's Spots
Measles

White spots with red areolae on buccal mucosa opposite molar teeth.
Appear in catarrhal stage before appearance of the rash.

Kussmaul's Respiration
Metabolic Acidosis.

Hyperventilation due to acidosis in diabetic ketoacidosis or in reneal failure.

Kussmaul's Sign
Constrictive Pericarditis. COAD

Paradoxical rise in jugular venous pressure on inspiration.

Kveim Test
Sarcoidosis

Granuloma formed in skin after intradermal injection of Kveim antigen - (extract from sarcoid lymph node).

Lachman Test
Instability Knee Joint

Flex knee to 20°.
Grasp both thigh and upper leg.
There should be no gliding at joint surfaces.
May be carried out with patient lying prone.

Larrey's Sign
Sacroiliac Disease

Patient, sitting in arm chair, raises himself on his arms, then allows himself to drop back on to the seat.
Jarring pain in SI joints.

Lasegue's Sign
Spinal Nerve Root Pressure

Limitation of flexion at the hip in straight leg raising.

Leser-Trelat Sign
Malignancy

Sudden eruption of multiple seborrheic keratoses.
Thought to indicate some hidden malignancy.
No longer thought authentic.

Lewis Triple Response
Normal Skin Response

Stroke skin with blunt object.
Redline within 15 seconds (local histamine reaction independent of nerve supply).

Spreading erythema (axon reflex via sensory nerves).
Wheal within several minutes (local urticaria from capillary fluid outflow).

L'hermitte's Sign
Demyelination Posterior Spinal Columns

Flex the neck.
Tingling electric sensations down spine towards legs.

Looser Sign
Osteomalacia

Radiological sign.
Thin transverse band of rarefaction in otherwise normal looking bone.

McBurney's Sign
Acute Appendicitis

Maximum tenderness elicited by finger tip pressure over McBurney's point.

McCarthy Reflex
Facial Palsy

Tap the supraorbital ridge.
Eye closes in lesions above the facial nucleus.
No effect in lesions at or below the nucleus.

McMurray's Sign
Torn Medial Meniscus

Flex the knee.
Slowly extend while also abducting and externally rotating leg.
Characteristic click as torn portion of meniscus is trapped momentarily between the condyles.

Milian's Sign
Facial Erysipelas

Skin infection spreads into pinna of ear.
Compare with subcutaneous cellulitis which stops short at pinna.

Moebius's Sign
Exophthalmos

Difficulty in ocular convergence when looking at near object.

Mongolian Blue Spots
Normality

Appear in babies over sacrum and lower back.
Common in deeply pigmented skin.
May be mistaken for bruises.
Become less obvious with age.

Moon's Molar
Congenital Syphilis

Small distorted cusps on the sixth year molars.

Moro Reflex
(Startle Reflex.)
Cerebral Abnormality in the Newborn

Response to startle in neonates.
Normal response is abduction and extension of the arms followed by flexion.
Abnormal response - thighs flex and arms extend.
Persistence beyond age of 8 to 10 weeks suspicious of cerebral palsy.
Unilateral response suggests brachial plexus injury or hemisphere lesion.

Moschowitz Sign
Peripheral Vascular Disease

Raise leg and apply tourniquet for five minutes.
Lower leg and remove tourniquet.
Delay of hyperaemia over few seconds indicates vascular insufficiency.

Murphy's Sign
Cholecystitis

The examiner's left hand is placed over the lower right ribs anteriorly with the thumb over the ninth costal cartilage and fundus of the gall bladder.
Patient "catches his breath" on deep inspiration.

Nelaton's Line
Congenital Dislocation of Hip

Draw a line from ischial tuberosity to anterior superior iliac spine. Normally tip of greater trochanter should lie below this line.

Ochsner Test
Median Nerve Palsy

Clasp hands firmly together. Injured finger does not flex.

Oppenheim's Sign
Pyramidal Tract Lesion

Extensor response, similar to Babinski, on stroking firmly down the inner aspect of the tibia.

Ortolani's Test
Congenital Dislocation of the Hip

A clunk is felt as head reduces on full abduction (cf Barlow's test).

Osler's Nodes
Subacute Bacterial Endocarditis

Transient, tender swellings in the pulps of fingers and toes. May be associated with "splinter haemorrhages" under the nails.

Pardee's Sign
Myocardial Infarct

Elevated S-T segment on ECG few hours after myocardial infarct.

Perkin's Line
Congenital Dislocation of Hip

Vertical radiological line dropped from outer edge of acetabulum (v. Hilgenreiner's line).
Femoral head should lie within this line.

Pethes' Test
Varicose Veins

Patient stands with veins distended.
Compress with finger tip suspected site of incompetence.
Patient rises on toes three times with compression maintained.
Positive result when veins empty only to refill promptly on releasing compression.

Phalen Sign
Carpal Tunnel Syndrome

Prolonged flexion of the wrist gives paraesthesiae over median nerve distribution.

Potter Facies
Various Syndromes

Low set ears.
Flattened nose.
Wide set eyes.

Queckenstedt Test
Patency of Subarachnoid Space

Compress the internal jugular vein during lumbar puncture.
Immediate rise in cerebrospinal fluid pressure indicates patent subarachnoid space.

Rinne Test
Deafness

Comparison between air and bone (mastoid) conduction
Normally, air is better than bone.
Rinne positive - air better than bone - normal ears and sensorineural deafness.
Rinne negative - bone better than air - confirmed by applying Barany noise box to opposite ear - conductive hearing loss.

Rockey's Sign
Depressed Malar Bone

Deviation of straight edged ruler, compared with the other side, when placed between malar prominence and external angular process.

Romana's Sign
Chaga's Disease

Unilateral closure of an eye due to firm red swelling in early stages of Trypanosoma cruzi infection.
Particularly in young children.

Romberg's Sign
Posterior Spinal Column Lesion

Patient stands with feet together.
Loss of balance on closing eyes.
Sign of sensory neuropathy.
Best seen in tabes dorsalis.
Not a test of cerebellar function.

Roth's Spots
Subacute Bacterial Endocarditis

Retinal signs of small emboli.

Rovsing's Sign
Acute Appendicitis

Manual pressure in the left iliac fossa gives pain in right iliac fossa.
Caused by gaseous back pressure in colon distending the caecum.

Saegesser's Sign
Ruptured Spleen

Pressure over the "splenic point", i.e. between sternomastoid and scalenus medius on the left side, causes pain.
Indicative of splenic rupture, even intracapsular haemorrhages.

Saint's Triad
Cholecystitis

Gall stones, hiatus hernia and diverticulitis.
Said to coexist frequently.

Schmalz Test
(v. Weber Test.)

Shenton's Line
Displaced Femoral Head

Radiological sign.
Continuation of line drawn along upper border of obturator foramen should run on along inferior surface of femoral head and neck.
Any gap indicates upward displacement of femoral head.

Signe de Crochet
Suppurative Tenosynovitis

Flexion of fingers in infection of digital tendon sheaths.

Signe de Dance
Intussusception

Feeling of emptiness in the right iliac fossa.

Sister (Marie) Joseph's Nodule
Intra-abdominal Malignancy

Hard subcutaneous nodule in umbilical region.
Signifies intra-abdominal malignancy, usually gastric or ovarian.

Stellwag's Sign
Exophthalmic Goitre

Retraction of upper eyelids due to spasm of levator palpebrae superioris.
Infrequent blinking and incomplete closure.

Thomas Test
Hip Joint Disease

Flex both knees up to chest.
Hold unaffected leg in this position.
Bring affected leg down to maximum extension.
Incomplete extension is measure of flexion contracture at the hip joint.

Thompson Test
Ruptured Achilles Tendon

Lay patient prone with knee flexed to 90^0.
Squeeze soleus-gastrocnemius muscle group.
Normally foot plantar flexes.
Fails to plantar flex if Achilles tendon ruptured.

Tinel's Sign
Nerve Regeneration

Tapping a nerve below the trauma site causes distal paraesthesiae.

Tinel's Sign
Carpal Tunnel Syndrome

Tapping over carpal tunnel produces paraesthesia over median nerve distribution.

Traube's Sign
Aortic Incompetence

Staccato murmur over femoral arteries.

Trendelenberg Sign
Congenital Dislocation of the Hip

When normal child stands on one leg, opposite buttock rises when viewed from behind.
When child stands on leg with dislocated hip, opposite buttock tends to drop.
In bilateral dislocations, there is a waddling gait.

Trendelenberg Test
Venous Valvular Incompetence

Patient lies supine.
The leg is elevated to empty the veins.
With the leg still elevated, pressure is applied over the saphenous opening in the groin.
Patient stands erect with pressure maintained.
Any filling of distal veins indicates incompetent deep vein valves.

Troisier's Sign
Gastric Carcinoma

Palpable lymph node (Virchow's node) in left supraclavicular fossa.

Trousseau's Sign
Tetany

Inflate a sphygmomanometer cuff above the arterial systolic pressure.
Spasm of forearm muscles occurs in cases of latent tetany producing 'main d'accoucheur'.

Trousseau's Sign
Carcinoma Pancreas

Fleeting thrombophlebitis.
Sign of carcinoma - usually pancreatic.
Manifestation of D.I.C. (Disseminated Intravascular Coagulation).

Uhthoff's Phenomenon
Multiple Sclerosis

Development, recrudescence or worsening of symptoms caused by any pyrexia.

von Graefe's Sign
Exophthalmic Goitre

"Lid lag" as upper eyelid lags behind on looking down.
Present in mild degrees of exophthalmos.

Weber Test
(Schmalz Test.)
Deafness

In unilateral disease.
Place vibrating tuning fork on mid line of vertex.
Conductive deafness - sound heard in bad ear.
Sensorineural deafness - sound heard in normal ear.

Westermark's Sign
Pulmonary Embolus

Radiological sign.
Diminished pulmonary vascular markings at site of pulmonary infarct.
Plain chest X-ray after infarct usually normal.

Wilson's Sign
Osteochondritis Dissecans

Best shortly after acute attack.
Patient is supine.
Flex affected knee to 90°.
Fully internally rotate and extend.
Pain over medial femoral condyle occurs 30° short of full extension.
Pain relieved by lateral rotation.

Glossary

Acalculia	Impaired arithmetic skills.
Achalasia of the cardia	Inability of oesophagus to relax.
Achlorhydria	Absence of normal gastric hydrochloric acid.
Acholuric	Absence of bile in the urine.
Acidosis	Respiratory or metabolic disturbance of body acid-base balance towards acid.
Acrocephaly	High, wide, short skull.
Aganglionosis	Absence of autonomic ganglion cells.
Agenesis	Failure to develop.
Agnosia	Inability to interpret visual, auditory and tactile stimuli.
Agraphia	Failure to express oneself in writing.
Alkalosis	Disturbance of body acid-base balance with arterial pH greater than 7.45.
Alopecia	Loss of hair.
Amaurotic	Unable to see. Blind.
Amenorrhoea	Absence of menstrual bleeding.
Amniocentesis	Transabdominal aspiration of amniotic fluid for analysis, abortion or radiography.
Amyloid	Infiltration of organs by waxy material in long term chronic infections.
Anaphylaxis	Exaggerated allergic response in someone previously sensitised.
Angiokeratoma	Benign, vascular, warty skin tumour.
Angioma	Benign vascular or lymphatic tumour.
Anhidrosis	Absence of sweating.
Anisocoria	Unequal pupils.
Anisocytosis	Variation in size of red blood cells.
Ankylosing	Joint stiffening.
Anosmia	Loss of sense of smell.
Aphasia	Difficulty with spoken word, either sensory (receptive) or motor (expressive).
Aphthous	Painful, superficial ulceration.

Apnoea	Cessation of breathing.
Aponeurosis	Broad tendinous sheath.
Apophysis	Bony outgrowth usually with muscular attachment.
Arachnodactyly	Long spidery fingers.
Areflexia	Absence of reflexes.
Arrhythmia	Irregular heart beat.
Arthralgia	Painful joints.
Arthropathy	Joint disease.
Ascites	Abnormal collection of peritoneal fluid.
Astrocytoma	Brain tumour, usually slow growing.
Ataxia	Unsteady gait.
Atherosclerosis	Arterial degeneration including lipid deposition, fibrosis and calcification.
Athetosis	Slow, writhing involuntary movements.
Atopic	Hypersensitivity to some common allergens.
Atresia	Congenital occlusion of some hollow organ.
Auerbach's plexus	Autonomic nerve plexus between muscle layers of gastro-intestinal tract.
Autosome	Any chromosome other than sex or accessory.
Blepharochalasia	Enlarged upper eyelids.
Blepharospasm	Involuntary closure of eyes.
Bony trabeculae	Mesh of strain resisting bony strands.
Brachycephaly	Short skull.
Brachydactyly	Short stubby fingers.
Bradycardia	Slow pulse rate.
Bruit	Murmur arising from blood vessel.
Buccal	Of the cheek.
Calcaneus	Heel bone, the largest tarsal bone.
Carcinoma in situ	Localised malignancy without penetration of epithelial basement membrane.
Cardiomegaly	Enlarged heart.
Cardiomyopathy	Diseased heart muscle.
Carpus	Small bones of hand.

Cellulitis	Diffuse acute infection of subcutaneous connective tissue.
Cerebellar ataxia	Unsteady gait due to cerebellar disease.
Cholangitis	Infection of bile duct system.
Chorda tympani	Nerve carrying sense of taste from anterior two thirds of tongue.
Choreiform	Involuntary movements resembling those of chorea.
Choreoathetosis	Involuntary movements resembling both chorea and athetosis.
Cirrhosis	Diffuse liver scarring with regeneration.
Clonus	Repetitive muscle contraction induced by sudden stretching.
Coloboma	Developmental eye defect.
Conductive deafness	Defect in external or middle ear.
Confabulation	Fabrication compensating for memory loss.
Coprolalia	Obscene utterings.
Cortisol	Adrenal cortical steroid hormone.
Coxa plana	Flattened femoral head.
Cranial sutures	Lines of apposition between individual cranial bones.
Cryptorchidism	Bilateral undescended testes.
Cubitus valgus	Increased carrying angle at elbow.
Cyanosis	Blue discolouration of skin and mucosae.
Demyelinating	Pathological loss of nerve sheath.
Dialysis	Artificial filtration of waste products in renal failure.
Diaphysis	Shaft of long bone.
Diastasis	A separation or parting.
Diencephalic	Relating to thalamus and hypothalamus.
Diplopia	Double vision.
Diverticulum	Localised protrusion of hollow viscus.
Dysarthria	Impaired speech due to neuromuscular disorder.
Dyskinesia	Difficulty in making purposeful movement.
Dysmorphism	Abnormality of shape or size.

Dysostosis	Faulty ossification of foetal cartilage.
Dyspareunia	Painful sexual intercourse.
Dysphagia	Difficulty in swallowing.
Dysplastic	Incomplete development or atypical cellular structure possibly predisposing to malignancy.
Dyspnoea	Shortness of breath.
Dystonia	Abnormality of muscle tone.
Dystrophy	Degenerative disorder due to imperfect nutrition.
Ecchymoses	Subcutaneous bruising.
Echocardiography	Heart scan using ultrasound.
Echolalia	Repetition of words spoken by others.
Electromyograph	Measurement of electrical activity during muscle contraction.
Encephalitis	Inflammation of the brain.
Endocardium	The lining of the heart chambers.
Enophthalmos	Sunken eyes.
Enteropathy	Bowel disease.
Ephelids	Freckles.
Epicanthic	Crescentic skin fold inner margin of eye.
Epiphysis	The growing end of a long bone.
Epistaxis	Nose bleed.
Epithelioma	Tumour of epithelium, most commonly squamous cell carcinoma.
Erysipelas	Haemolytic streptococcal skin infection, commonly on the face.
Erythroblast	Nucleated precursor to mature red blood cell.
Erythrocyte	Red blood cell.
Erythropoiesis	Formation of red blood cells.
ESR	Erythrocyte sedimentation rate.
Exfoliation	Falling away of dead tissue from skin.
Exophthalmos	Protruding eyes.
Fasciculation	Localised involuntary muscle twitching.

Medical Eponyms

Festination	Uncontrolled acceleration.
Fibrillation	Incoordinated muscle contraction most commonly seen in heart.
Fibroadenosis	Benign proliferation of fibrous and glandular breast tissue.
Fistula	Abnormal communication between two hollow organs or between skin and hollow organ.
Flaccid	Limp. Lacking muscle tone.
Foramen	Opening.
Galactorrhoea	Pathological lactation in either sex.
Gallup rhythm	Three heart sounds instead of usual two.
Genu valgum	Knock knees.
Genu varus	Bowleg or bandy legged.
Glabella	Midpoint between supraorbital ridges.
Glenoid	Shallow cavity in shoulder blade as part of shoulder joint.
Glomerulonephritis	Acute, subacute or chronic inflammation of vascular tuft forming kidney filtration unit.
Glossoptosis	Tongue falls backwards and downwards.
Granuloma	Mass of chronic inflammatory cells.
Gynaecomastia	Enlargement of male breast.
Haemangioblastoma	Vascular tumour of central nervous system.
Haemangioma	Benign tumour of blood vessels.
Haemarthrosis	Bleeding into a joint.
Haematuria	Blood in the urine.
Haemolysis	Red cell destruction.
Haemoptysis	To cough up blood.
Haemosiderosis	Abnormal deposition of iron in organs.
Hemiplegia	Paralysis one side of body.
Hepatomegaly	Enlarged liver.
Hepatosplenomegaly	Enlarged liver and spleen.
Hirsutism	Male distribution of hair in women.
Histiocyte	A cell involved in host protection mechanisms.

Hydrocephalus	Abnomally large amount of intracranial cerebrospinal fluid.
Hyperacusis	Abnormally acute hearing.
Hyperaesthesia	Exaggerated sensitivity to external stimuli.
Hyperbilirubinaemia	Abnormally high blood level of bile pigment.
Hyperchromatic	Increased affinity to staining with dyes.
Hyperkalaemia	Abnormally high blood level of potassium.
Hyperkeratosis	Excessively thick horny layer of skin.
Hyperkinesis	Abnormally intense, agitated motor activity.
Hyperlipidaemia	Abnormally high blood level of lipids.
Hyperplasia	Benign cellular proliferation in response to specific cause.
Hyperreflexia	Exaggerated reflexes.
Hypertelorism	Abnormal distance between paired organs e.g. eyes.
Hypertonia	Increased muscle tone.
Hypoglycaemia	Abnormally low blood sugar level.
Hypogonadism	The secondary sexual consequences of deficient production of sex hormones by gonads.
Hyponatraemia	Abnormally low blood level of sodium.
Hypospadias	Congenital defect of penile urethra.
Hypotension	Low blood pressure.
Hypothenar	Prominence at inner border of palm caused by intrinsic muscles of the little finger.
Hypotonia	Reduced muscle tone.
Hypovolaemia	Abnormal reduction in circulating blood volume.
Iatrogenic	Resulting from therapy.
Ichthyosis	Fish scale skin.
Immunoglobulin	Protein with antibody capability.
Impetigo	Contagious pustular skin disease.
Indolent ulcer	Painless ulcer, slow to heal.
Infarct	Area of dead tissue, usually wedge shaped, due to occluded blood supply.
Intermittent claudication	Muscle cramps due to deficient blood supply.
Intra-epidermal carcinoma	Non-invasive skin cancer.

Intussusception	Telescoping of one section of bowel into its neighbour.
Iridocyclitis	Inflammation of iris and ciliary body.
Ischaemia	Impaired blood supply.
Kernicterus	Cerebral damage due to prolonged jaundice.
Koilonychia	Spoon shaped finger nails.
Kyphosis	Excessive forwards flexion of thoracic spine.
Labium majus	Outer margin of female genitalia.
Labrum	Brim to joint cavity e.g glenoid in shoulder.
Lentigines	Small dark brown spots.
Leucodystrophy	Disorder of myelin metabolism.
Leucopenia	Abnormally low blood white cell count.
Leukaemia	Malignant disease of white blood cells.
Leukoerythroblastic	Immature white and red blood cells in circulation.
Lipomatosis	Multiple benign fatty tumours.
Lower motor neurone	Nerve from cranial motor nucleus or spinal cord to muscle.
Lumbar lordosis	Abnormally marked anterior curvature of lumbar spine.
Lymphadenopathy	Disease of lymph glands.
Lymphoedema	Swelling due to lymphatic obstruction.
Lymphoma	Malignant tumour of lymph glands.
Lymphopenia	Abnormally few circulating lymphocytes.
Macrocephaly	Large head.
Macrocytosis	Abnormally large red corpuscular volume.
Macroglobulinaemia	Increased circulating level of globulin.
Macroglossia	Enlarged tongue.
Macrophage	Cell, found in many tissues, involved in host protection mechanisms.
Macrosomia	Gigantism.
Macrotia	Abnormally large ears.
Macula (lutea)	Yellowish spot in central retina where visual acuity is greatest.

Medical Eponyms

Macule	Circumscribed area of discoloured skin.
Malleolus	Bony point each side of ankle joint.
Mastoiditis	Infection of bony mastoid process behind ear.
Megaloblast	Abnormally large nucleated red blood cell precursor seen in bone marrow.
Melanoma	Benign or malignant tumour of melanocytes.
Meningioma	Typically benign tumour of membranes covering the brain.
Menorrhagia	Excessive menstruation.
Mesonephron	Stage of kidney development leaving vestigial remnants only in the adult.
Metacarpus	Five long bones betweeen carpus and phalanges.
Mataphysis	Actively growing end of long bone adjacent to epiphyseal cartilage.
Metastasis	Distant tumour spread.
Metatarsus	Five long bones between tarsus and phalanges.
Microcephaly	Small head.
Micrognathia	Receding chin.
Microphthalmia	Abnormally small eyes.
Microtia	Abnormally small ears.
Miosis	Marked constriction of pupil.
Mononucleosis	Abnormally high level of circulating mononuclear cells.
Myalgia	Painful muscles.
Myasthenia	Weak, abnormally fatigued muscles.
Myelin sheath	Insulating sheath around nerve fibres.
Myeloid	Pertaining to bone marrow.
Myocarditis	Inflammatory disease of heart muscle.
Myoclonus	Brief contraction of single muscle or muscle group.
Myoglobinuria	Myoglobin excretion in urine following extensive muscle damage.
Myxoedema	Symptom complex resulting from underactive thyroid gland.
Myxoma	Benign but infiltrating tumour of unknown origin.

Naevus	Classically any congenital skin blemish but more loosely applied to any pigmented skin tumour.
Necrolysis	Separation of dead tissue from normal.
Necrosis	Changes that follow cell death.
Neoplasm	New growth.
Nephropathy	Kidney disease.
Neural crest	Embryonic structure thought to give rise to cerebral, spinal and autonomic ganglia.
Neuralgia	Pain in area supplied by individual sensory nerve.
Neuroblastoma	Highly malignant tumour (adrenal medulla and sympathetic chain) in children.
Neuroectodermal	Related to cells from embryonic neural crest.
Neurofibrils	Fine threads within the neurone.
Neuroma	Benign tumour of nerve.
Neuropathy	Diseased nerves.
Neutropenia	Decreased number of circulating neutrophils.
Nystagmus	Rapid, rhythmic movements of the eye.
Oedema	Swelling due to excessive tissue fluid.
Oligohydramnios	Reduced amount of amniotic fluid.
Oliguria	Abnormally small urinary output.
Omphalocele	Herniation into the umbilical cord.
Ophthalmoplegia	Paralysis of ocular muscles.
Opisthotonus	Arching of body due to strong spinal muscle contraction.
Osteochondritis	Inflammatory disease of bone and adjoining cartilage.
Osteogenesis	Bone formation.
Osteoma	Benign tumour of bone.
Osteomalacia	Softened, deformed bones due to defective mineralisation.
Osteomyelitis	Bacterial infection of bone.
Osteoporosis	Deterioration in bone structure due to mineral and protein loss.

Medical Eponyms

Palilalia	Repetition of own words.
Pancytopenia	Reduced circulating numbers of all forms of blood cells.
Papilloedema	Swollen optic disc due to raised intracranial pressure.
Papule	Palpable skin lesion.
Paraesthesia	Skin sensations e.g. 'pins and needles' without external stimulus.
Parasympathetic system	Part of autonomic nervous system.
Parathyroid	Four glands situated two each side of thyroid gland.
Parenchyma	The functioning element of any gland or organ.
Paronychia	Infection in nail fold.
Pathognomonic	Diagnostic.
Perfusion	Passage of blood or other fluid through an organ.
Pericarditis	Inflammation of sac enveloping the heart.
Perifollicular	Skin changes around a hair follicle.
Peyer's patches	Collections of lymphoid tissue in wall of terminal ileum.
Phaeochromocytoma	Benign adrenal medullary tumour secreting hormone that raises blood pressure.
Phagocytosis	Means by which white blood cells engulf bacteria or foreign body.
Phalanx	Individual long bone in a digit.
Photophobia	Visual hypersensitivity to light.
Pingueculae	Pigmented scleral thickenings.
Plasma cells	Synthesize and secrete immunoglobulins.
Platelet	Cellular fragment circulating in great numbers with important role in clotting process.
Pneumothorax	Air in pleura causing lung collapse.
Poikilocyte	Irregularly shaped red blood cell.
Poliosis	Whitening of ends of eye lashes.
Polycythaemia	Abnormally large number of circulating red blood cells.
Polydactyly	More than normal number of digits or parts of digits.
Pons	Part of brain stem.

Medical Eponyms

Popliteal	Pertaining to the region behind the knee.
Portal circulation	Venous drainage of the gastro-intestinal tract.
Portal hypertension	Abnormally high pressure within portal venous system.
Post herpetic	Following shingles.
Proprioceptive	Aware of movement or position of body or body parts.
Proptosis	Protruding eyes.
Proteinuria	Protein excreted in the urine.
Pruritis	Itching sensation.
Pseudobulbar palsy	Difficulty in swallowing or speaking due to upper motor neurone lesion.
Ptosis	Prolapse of an organ, most commonly drooping upper eyelid.
Purpura	Widespread focal haemorrhages into the skin.
Radial styloid	Bony prominence upper outer aspect of wrist joint.
Renal glomerulus	Vascular tuft essential to renal filtration process.
Schirrous	Hard, gritty tumour.
Sclerodactyly	Atrophic tapering of fingers distal to proximal interphalangeal joints.
Scleroderma	Localised or generalised skin hardening.
Scoliosis	Lateral curvature of spine.
Scotoma	Blind spot.
Sensorineural deafness	Defect in cochlea or its neural connection to brain.
Sequestrum	Necrotic tissue separated from viable tissue, commonly seen in osteomyelitis.
Simian	Ape like.
Situs inversus	Horizontal transposition of organs.
Spherocytosis	Spherical red blood cells rather than normal biconcave disc shape.
Spherophakia	Spherical ocular lens.
Splenomegaly	Enlarged spleen.
Spondylitis	Inflammation of one or more vertebrae.
Steatorrhoea	Excessively fatty stools.

Medical Eponyms

Stomatitis	Infection of the mouth.
Strabismus	Squint.
Strangulation	Impairment of blood supply, usually relating to bowel in a hernia.
Striae	Narrow lines or streaks.
Stroma	Supporting framework within an organ.
Subluxation	Incomplete joint dislocation.
Sympathetic system	Part of the autonomic nervous system.
Syncope	A fainting attack.
Syndactyly	Fusion or webbing between adjoining digits.
Synophrys	Confluent eyebrows
Synostosis	Fusion between adjoining bones.
Synovium	Lining membrane in joint, tendon sheath or bursa.
Tachycardia	Increased heart rate.
Tarsus	Small bones between ankle and metatarsals.
Telangiectasis	Collection of small vessels; arterial, venous, capillary or lymphatic.
Tenosynovitis	Inflammation of tendon sheaths.
Tetany	Muscular spasms due to hyperexcitability caused by low serum calcium.
Thenar	Group of intrinsic muscles of the thumb.
Thrombocytopenia	Deficiency of circulating blood platelets.
Thrombophlebitis	Inflammatory clotting in veins.
Thrombosis	Intravascular blood clotting.
Thyroglobulin	Thyroid gland protein converting to thyroxine.
Tic	Abrupt, aimless muscle contraction, usually facial.
Tinnitus	Various noises heard subjectively within the ear or head.
Tophus	Urate deposits in ear lobes of gouty patients.
Transcoelomic	Across body cavities; peritoneal, pleural, pericardial.
Transitional epithelium	Epithelium undergoing change from one form to another.
Trichophyton	Ringworm fungus.

Medical Eponyms

Trigonocephaly	Triangular shaped head.
Trophic	Changes due to nutritional deficiency.
Trypanosomiasis	Group of diseases caused by infection with Trypanosoma.
Tylosis	Thickened skin palms and soles.
Upper motor neurone	Nerve connecting motor area of cerebral cortex to cranial motor nucleus or spinal cord.
Uraemia	Symptom complex due to kidney failure.
Uveitis	Inflammation of uveal tract within the eye.
Vacuoles	Clear spaces within a cell's cytoplasm.
Vasculitis	Inflammation of blood vessels.
Vertigo	Giddiness, particularly rotational.
Vesicle	Small blister like swelling.
Virilism	Male secondary sexual characteristics in a female.
Vitiligo.	Patchy loss of skin pigmentation.
Xanthelasma	Localised cholesterol deposits at inner margin of eyelids.
Xanthochromia	Yellow colouring in cerebrospinal fluid.
Xanthoma	Localised collection of lipid in the skin or tendons.
Xerostoma	Dry mouth.

References

A Psychiatric Catechism. Peter McGuffin. Steven Greer.
Aston's Short Textbook of Orthopaedics and Trauma.
Davidson's Principles and Practice of Medicine.
Encyclopaedia Britannica.
E. Noble Chamberlain's Symptoms and Signs in Clinical Medicine.
Essential Paediatrics. David Hull. Derek I. Johnston.
Essential Surgical Practice. A.Cushieri. G.R.Giles. A.R.Moossa.
General Pathology. J.B.Walter. M.S.Israel.
Hamilton Bailey's Physical Signs in Clinical Surgery.
Hutchinson's Clinical Methods. Michael Swash. Stuart Mason.
Illingworth and Dick's Surgical Pathology.
Lecture Notes on Diseases of the Ear, Nose and Throat. P.D. Bull.
Lecture Notes on Haematology. N.C. Hughes-Jones.
Notes on Psychiatry. I.M. Ingram. G.C. Timbury. R.M. Mowbray.
Oxford Handbook of Clinical Specialties. J.A.B.Collier. J.M.Longmore.
The A-Z Reference Book of Syndromes and Inherited Disorders. Patricia Gilbert.
Undergraduate Obstetrics and Gynaecology. M.G.R.Hull. D.N.Joyce. Gillian Turner.
Neurology - A Concise Clinical Text. Michael Swash. Martin S. Schwartz.
A Manual of Dermatology. Pillsbury and Heaton.
Essential Neurology. I.M.S. Wilkinson.
Essential Urology. Nigel Bullock. Gary Sibley. Robert Whitaker.
Practical Paediatric Problems. James H. Hutchison. Forrester Cockburn.
Lecture Notes on Geriatrics. Nicholas Coni. William Davison. Stephen Webster.
UCH Textbook of Psychiatry. Heinz Wolff. Anthony Bateman. David Sturgeon.
Modern Obstetrics in General Practice. G.N. Marsh.
Dictionary of Medical Eponyms. B.G. Firkin. J.A. Whitworth.
The Oxford Textbook of Surgery.
Churchill's Medical Dictionary.
Clinical Ophthalmology. Jack J. Kanski.

Apley's System of Orthopaedics and Fractures. A. Graham Apley.
   Louis Solomon.
Neurological Differential Dignosis. John Patten.
Clinical Otolaryngology. E.G.D. Maran. P.M. Stell.
An Atlas of Clinical Syndromes. H.R. Wiedemann. J. Kunze.
   H. Dibbern.

Index

Achard-Thiers Syndrome 93
Acquired Immunity Deficiency
  Syndrome 93
Adair-Dighton Syndrome 93
Adam's Syndrome 94
Addison's Anaemia 1
Addison's Disease 1
Addison-Schilder's Disease 2
Adie Pupil 193
Adrenogenital Syndrome 94
Adson's Syndrome 94
Adson Test 193
Ahumada-del Castillo
  Syndrome 94
Aicardi's Syndrome 95
Albers-Schonberg Disease 2
Albright's Hereditary
  Osteodystrophy 2
Albright Syndrome 95
Alder's Sign 193
Allen Test 194
Allis Sign 194
Alpers Syndrome 95
Alport Syndrome 96
Alstrom Syndrome 96
Alzheimer's Disease 3
Andersen's Disease 3
Angelman's Syndrome 96
Aniridia-Wilms Tumour 3
Aortic Arch Syndrome 96
Apert's Syndrome 97
Apley's Test 194
Argyll Robertson Sign 195
Arnold-Chiari Syndrome 97
Ascher's Syndrome 97

Aschoff Nodule 195
Askin Tumour 3
Asperger's Syndrome 98
Assman Focus 4
Austin Flint Murmur 195
Australia Antigen 4
Avellis Syndrome 98

Babinski's "Rising up" Sign 195
Babinski's Sign 196
Bainbridge Reflex 196
Baker's Cyst 4
Ballance's Sign 196
Bankart Lesion 4
Banti's Syndrome 98
Bardet-Biedl Syndrome 98
Barlow's Disease 4
Barlow's Test 196
Barlow Syndrome 99
Barrett's Oesophagus 5
Bartholin's Cyst 5
Barton's Fracture 5
Bartter Syndrome 99
Basedow's Disease 5
Batten's Disease 5
Batten-Vogt Syndrome 99
Battered Baby Syndrome 99
Battle's Sign 196
Baumann's Angle 197
Baumgarten Syndrome 100
Bazin's Disease 6
Beau's Lines 197
Becker's Muscular Dystrophy 7
Becker's Syndrome 100
Beck's Triad 197

241

Beckwith-Weidman
   Syndrome 100
Behcet's Disease 7
Bell's Palsy 7
Bell's Reflex 197
Benedikt's Syndrome 100
Bennett's Fracture 8
Berger Disease 8
Bernard-Soulier Syndrome 101
Bernstein's Test 197
Berry's Sign 198
Bezold's Abscess 8
Bietti's Nodular Dystrophy 8
Binswanger's Encephalopathy 9
Bird Fancier's Lung 9
Bishop's Score 198
Bitot's Spots 198
Bland-White-Garland
   Syndrome 101
Blind Loop Syndrome 101
Bloom's Syndrome 101
Blue Diaper Syndrome 102
Boas Sign 198
Bochdalek Hernia 9
Bockhart's Impetigo 9
Boerhaave Syndrome 102
Bonnevie-Ullrich Syndrome 102
Bornholm Disease 9
Bouchard's Nodes 199
Bourneville's Disease 10
Bowen's Disease 10
Brandt's Syndrome 102
Branham's Sign 199
Brenner Tumour 10
Bright's Disease 11
Briquet's Syndrome 102
Brill's Disease 11
Brissaud-Sicard Syndrome 103
Broadbent Sign 199

Brock Syndrome 103
Brodie's Abscess 11
Brodie's Serocystic Sarcoma 12
Brodie-Trendelenberg Test 199
Brown-Sequard Syndrome 103
Brudzinski's Sign 199
Brun's Frontal Ataxia 12
Brushfield Spots 200
Bruton's
   Agammaglobulinaemia 12
Buchanan's Syndrome 104
Budd-Chiari Syndrome 104
Buerger's Disease 12
Burkitt's Tumour 13
Burning Feet Syndrome 104
Burton Line 200
Buruli Ulcer 13
Buschke-Loewenstein
   Tumours 14
Bywaters Syndrome 104

Cafe-au-lait Spots 200
Caffey's Disease (Syndrome) 14
Caisson Disease 14
Campbell de Morgan Spots 200
Camurati's Disease 15
Canavan's Disease 15
Cantrell's Syndrome 104
Capgras Syndrome 105
Caplan's Syndrome 105
Caput Medusae 200
Carcinoid Syndrome 105
Carini's Syndrome 106
Caroli's Disease 15
Carpal Tunnel Syndrome 106
Carrion's Disease 16
Carr's Concretions 16
Carvallo's Sign 200
Ceelen's Disease 16

Cervical Rib Syndrome 106
Cestan-Chenais Syndrome 106
Chagas Disease 17
Charcot's Fever 17
Charcot's Joints 17
Charcot's Triad 201
Charcot-Marie-Tooth
  Syndrome 107
Chediak-Higashi Syndrome 107
Chevrier's Percussion Test 201
Cheyne-Stokes Respiration 201
Chiari-Frommel Syndrome 107
Chikungunya Fever 18
Chimney Sweep's Cancer 18
Christensen-Krabbe Disease 18
Christmas Disease 18
Churg-Strauss Syndrome 108
Chvostek Sign 201
Clark's Naevus 19
Claude's Syndrome 108
Clay Shoveller's Disease 19
Clumsy Child Syndrome 108
Clutton's Joints 19
Coalition Syndrome 109
Coat's Disease 19
Cockayne Syndrome 109
Cock's Peculiar Tumour 20
Codman's Sign 202
Codman's Triangle 202
Coffin-Lowry Syndrome 109
Cogan's Syndrome 110
Colles Fracture 20
Collet-Sicard Syndrome 110
Conn's Syndrome 110
Conradi-Hunerman Syndrome 111
Cooley's Anaemia 20
Cori's Disease 21
Cornelia de Lange Syndrome 111
Coroli Syndrome 111

Corrigan's Pulse 202
Costen's Syndrome 112
Cotard's Syndrome 112
Courvoisier's Law 202
Couvade Syndrome 112
CREST Syndrome 112
Creutzfeldt-Jakob Disease 21
Cri-du chat Syndrome 113
Crigler-Najjar Syndrome 113
Crohn's Disease 21
Cronkhite-Canada Syndrome 113
Crouzon's Syndrome
  (Disease) 114
Crush Syndrome 114
Cruveilhier-Baumgarten
  Syndrome 114
Cruveilhier's Sign 202
Cubital Tunnel Syndrome 115
Cullen's Sign 203
Curling's Ulcer 22
Curtis-Fitz-Hugh Syndrome 115
Cushing's Disease 22
Cushing Reflex 203
Cushing's Syndrome 115
Cushing's Ulcer 23

da Costa Syndrome 116
Dalrymple's Sign 203
Dandy-Walker Syndrome 116
Darier's Sign 203
de Clerambault's Syndrome 116
Degos's Syndrome (Disease) 117
de Grouchy's Syndrome 117
Dejerine-Roussey Syndrome 117
Dejerine-Sottas Disease 23
Dejerine-Thomas Disease 23
Del Castillo Syndrome 118
de Quervain's Disease 24
de Quervain's Tenosynovitis 24

Dercum's Disease 24
Devic's Disease 25
Dhobi Itch 25
Diamond-Blackfan
 Syndrome 118
Dietl's Crisis 25
Di George Syndrome 118
Di Guglielmo's Disease 25
Down Syndrome 119
Drawer Test 203
Dresbach's Syndrome 119
Dressler's Syndrome 120
Duane's Retraction
 Syndrome 120
Dubin-Johnson Syndrome 120
Duchenne Muscular
 Dystrophy 26
Dugas's Sign 204
Duhring's Disease 27
Dumping Syndrome 120
Dupuytren's Contracture 27
Dysmnesic Syndrome 121

Eagle-Barrett Syndrome 121
Eales Disease 27
Eaton-Lambert Syndrome 121
Ebstein's Anomaly Syndrome 121
Eck Fistula 27
Edwards's Syndrome 122
Ehlers-Danlos Syndrome 122
Eight Day Disease 28
Eisenmenger Syndrome 122
Ekbom Syndrome 123
Ellis-van Creveld Syndrome 123
Engelmann's Syndrome 123
Epstein-Barr Virus 28
Epstein Syndrome 124
Erb's Muscular Dystrophy 28

Erb's Palsy 29
Erdheim's Cystic
 Medionecrosis 29
Ewing's Tumour 29

Fabry Disease 30
Fallot's Tetralogy 30
Fanconi Anaemia 31
Fanconi Syndrome 124
Farmer's Lung 31
Favre-Goldmann Syndrome 124
Fawn's Tail 204
Felty's Syndrome 124
Finkelstein's Test 204
Fisher Syndrome 125
Foetal Alcohol Syndrome 125
Forbes-Albright Syndrome 125
Fordyce's Disease 31
Forestier's Disease 32
Foster-Kennedy Syndrome 125
Fournier's Gangrene 32
Foville's Syndrome 126
Fragile X Syndrome 126
Francheschetti-Klein
 Syndrome 126
Fregoli Syndrome 127
Freiburg's Disease 32
Frey's Syndrome 127
Friedreich's Ataxia 32
Frohlich's Syndrome 127
Froin's Syndrome 127
Froment's Sign 204

Galeazzi Fracture 33
Galleazzi Sign 204
Gamstorp's Disease 33
Ganser's Syndrome 128
Gardner's Syndrome 128

Medical Eponyms

Garre's Disease 33
Gartner's Cyst 34
Gaucher's Disease 34
Gerstmann's Syndrome 128
Gerstmann-Straussler
 Syndrome 129
Ghon Focus 34
Gilbert's Syndrome 129
Gilles de la Tourette's
 Syndrome 129
Glanzmann's Thrombasthenia 35
Goldenhar Syndrome 129
Goodpasture's Syndrome 130
Goodsall's Rule 205
Good's Syndrome 130
Gordon's Sign 205
Gordon's Syndrome 130
Gorham's Disease 35
Gorlin's Syndrome 131
Gower Sign 205
Gradenigo's Syndrome 131
Graham Steel Murmur 205
Grave's Disease 35
Grawitz Tumour 36
Grey Baby Syndrome 131
Grey Turner's Sign 205
Gritti-Stokes Amputation 36
Gronblad-Strandberg
 Syndrome 131
Grumbach's Disease 36
Guillain-Barre Syndrome 132
Gunn's Pupil 206

Haemolytic-Uraemic
 Syndrome 132
Haglund Syndrome 132
Hallerman-Streiff-
 Francoise Syndrome 133
Hallevorden-Spatz Disease 37

Hallgren's Syndrome 133
Hamman's Sign 206
Hand-Foot Syndrome 133
Hand-Schuller-Christian
 Disease 37
Hangman's Fracture 37
Hanot's Cirrhosis 37
Hansen's Disease 38
Harrison's Sulci 206
Hartnup Disease 38
Hashimoto's Disease 39
Heberden's Nodes 207
Heerfordt's Syndrome 133
Henoch Schonlein Purpura 39
Hepato-renal Syndrome 133
Hers's Disease 40
Hess Test 207
Hilgenreiner's Line 207
Hirschprung's Disease 40
Hochsinger's Sign 207
Hodgkin's Lymphoma 40
Holmes-Adie Syndrome 134
Holt-Oram Syndrome 134
Homan's Sign 208
Horner's Syndrome 134
Horsley's Sign 208
Howell-Evans Syndrome 135
Howship-Romberg Sign 208
Humidifier Lung 41
Hungry Bones Syndrome 135
Hunner's Ulcer 41
Hunter's Syndrome 135
Huntington's Chorea 41
Hunt's Syndrome 136
Hurler's Syndrome 136
Hutchinson-Gilford Syndrome 136
Hutchinson's Freckle 42
Hutchinson's Sign
 (Herpes Zoster) 208

Medical Eponyms

Hutchinson's Sign (Middle
  Meningeal
  Haemorrhage) 208
Hutchinson's Teeth 209
Hutchinson's Triad 209
Hutchinson's Tumour 42
Hyperprolactinaemia
  Syndrome 137

Irritable Bowel Syndrome 137
Ivemark Syndrome 137

Jaccoud's Syndrome 138
Jacksonian Epilepsy 42
Jansen's Syndrome 138
Jefferson Fracture 42
Jendrassik's Manoeuvre 209
Job's Syndrome 138
Joffroy's Sign 209
Johansson-Larsen's Disease 43
Jones-Nevin Syndrome 138

Kallman's Syndrome 139
Kanavel's Sign 209
Kanner's Syndrome 139
Kantor's String Sign 210
Kaposi's Sarcoma 43
Kaposi's Varicelliform
  Eruption 43
Kartagener's Syndrome 139
Kasabach-Merritt Syndrome 139
Kast's Syndrome 139
Katayama Fever 43
Kawasaki Syndrome 139
Kearns-Sayre Syndrome 140
Kehr's Sign 210
Kenawy's Sign 210
Kernig's Sign 210

Kestenbaum's Sign 210
Kienbock's Disease 44
Kiloh-Nevin Syndrome 140
Kinnier-Wilson Disease 44
Kissing Disease 44
Kleine-Levin Syndrome 140
Klinefelter's Syndrome 141
Klippel-Feil Syndrome 141
Klippel-Trenaunay Syndrome 142
Klumpke's Paralysis 44
Kluver-Bucy Syndrome 142
Kocher's Sign 211
Kohler's Disease 44
Koplik's Spots 211
Korsakoff Syndrome 142
Krabbe's Disease 45
Krukenberg Tumour 45
Kugelberg-Welander Disease 45
Kummell's Disease 46
Kussmaul's Disease 46
Kussmaul's Respiration 211
Kussmaul's Sign 211
Kveim Test 211
Kyasanur Forest Disease 46

Lachman Test 212
Ladd's Bands 46
Laennec's Cirrhosis 46
Lambert's Syndrome 143
Lambert-Eaton Myasthenic
  Syndrome 143
LAMB Syndrome 143
Landouzy-Dejerine
  Dystrophy 47
Landry's Paralysis 47
Larrey's Sign 212
Larsen's Syndrome 143
Lasegue's Sign 212

Medical Eponyms

Lassa Fever 47
Lawrence-Moon-Biedl
   Syndrome 144
Leber's Hereditary Optic
   Atrophy 48
Lederer's Anaemia 48
Le Fort Fractures 48
Legg-Calve-Perthes' Disease 48
Legionnaire's Disease 49
Leigh's Disease 49
Lennert's Lymphoma 49
LEOPARD Syndrome 144
Leriche Syndrome 144
Leri's Disease 50
Lermoyez Syndrome 145
Lesch-Nyhan Syndrome 145
Leser-Trelat Sign 212
Letterer-Siwe Disease 50
Levy-Roussey Syndrome 145
Lewis Triple Response 212
Leydig Cell Tumour 50
L'hermitte's Sign 213
Libman-Sach's Endocarditis 51
Liddle's Syndrome 146
Littre's Hernia 51
Locked In Syndrome 146
Loeffler's Syndrome 146
Looser Sign 213
Lorain-Type Dwarfism 51
Lou Gehrig's Disease 51
Louis-Bar Syndrome 147
Lowe's Syndrome 147
Lucey-Driscoll Syndrome 148
Ludwig's Angina 52
Lutembacher's Syndrome 148
Luxury Perfusion Syndrome 148
Lyell's Disease 52
Lyme Disease 52
Lynch Type Tumours 52

MacLeod's Syndrome 148
Madelung's Deformity 53
Maffucci's Syndrome 149
Majocchi's Granuloma 53
Maladie de Reclus 53
Maladie de Roger 53
Mallory-Weiss Syndrome 149
Maltworker's Lung 54
Marburg Disease 54
Marchesani Syndrome 149
Marchiafava-Bignami Disease 54
Marcus Gunn Syndrome 149
Marfan's Syndrome 149
Marie and Sanger-Brown
   Syndrome 150
Marion's Disease 55
Marjolin's Ulcer 55
Maroteaux-Lamy Syndrome 150
Maydl's Hernia 55
McArdle's Disease 55
McBurney's Sign 213
McCarthy Reflex 213
McCune-Albright Syndrome 151
McMurray's Sign 214
Megacystitis Mega-Ureter
   Syndrome 151
Meibomian Cyst 56
Meig's Syndrome 151
Meige's Syndrome 151
Meleney's Burrowing Ulcer 56
Meleney's Postoperative
   Synergistic Gangrene 56
MEN 1 56
MEN 2 57
Mendelsohn's Syndrome 152
Menetrier's Disease 57
Meniere's Disease
   (Syndrome) 57
Menke's Syndrome 152

Mikulicz's Disease 58
Milian's Sign 214
Millard-Gubler Syndrome 152
Miller-Fisher Syndrome 153
Milroy's Disease 58
Minkowski-Chauffard
  Disease 59
Mirizzi's Syndrome 153
Moebius' Sign 214
Moebius' Syndrome 153
Mollaret's Meningitis 59
Monckeberg's Sclerosis 59
Mondor's Disease 59
Mongolian Blue Spots 214
Monteggia Fracture 60
Moon's Molar 214
Morgagni Hernia 60
Moro Reflex 215
Morquio's Syndrome 153
Morton's Metatarsalgia 60
Mounier-Kuhn Disease 60
Moschcowitz's Syndrome 154
Moschowitz Sign 215
Mule Spinner's Cancer 61
Munchausen Syndrome 154
Munchausen by Proxy
  Syndrome 155
Murphy's Sign 215
Murray Valley Fever 61

Naffziger Syndrome 155
Nail-Patella I Syndrome 155
NAME Syndrome 155
Nelaton's Line 216
Nelson's Syndrome 155
Nephrotic Syndrome 156
Nezelhof's Syndrome 156
Niemann-Pick Disease 61
Noonan's Syndrome 156

Norrie's Disease 62

Ochsner Test 216
Ogilvie's Syndrome 157
Oldfield's Syndrome 157
Ollier's Disease (Syndrome) 62
Omsk Haemorrhagic Fever 62
Ondine's Curse 62
One and a Half Syndrome 157
Oppenheim's Sign 216
Oroya Fever 63
Ortner's Syndrome 157
Ortolani's Test 216
Osgood-Schlatter's Disease 63
Osler-Rendu-Weber
  Syndrome 158
Osler's Disease 63
Osler's Nodes 216
Osler-Vaquez Disease 63
Othello Syndrome 158

Pacemaker Syndrome 158
Page Syndrome 158
Paget-Schroetter Syndrome 158
Paget's Disease of Bone 64
Paget's Disease of the Nipple 64
Paget's Recurring Fibroma 65
Pancoast Tumour (Syndrome) 65
Panner's Disease 65
Paraneoplastic Syndrome 159
Pardee's Sign 217
Parinaud's Syndrome 159
Parkes-Weber Syndrome 159
Parkinson's Disease 65
Parry's Disease 66
Patau's Syndrome 160
Paterson-Brown-Kelly
  Syndrome 160
Pel-Ebstein Fever 66

Pellegrini-Stieda Syndrome 160
Pendred's Syndrome 161
Pepper's Syndrome 161
Periodic Syndrome 161
Perkin's Line 217
Perthes' Disease 66
Pethes' Test 217
Peutz-Jeghers Syndrome 161
Peyronie's Disease 67
Pfeiffer Syndrome 162
Phalen Sign 217
Pick's Disease (Pericarditis) 68
Pick's Disease (Psychiatric) 67
Pickwickian Syndrome 162
Pierre-Robin Syndrome 162
Pink Disease 68
Plummer's Disease 68
Plummer-Vinson Syndrome 162
Poland's Syndrome 163
Pompe Disease 69
Posner-Schlossman
   Syndrome 163
Post Cholecystectomy
   Syndrome 163
Post Concussional Syndrome 163
Post Hepatitis Syndrome 164
Post Myocardial Infarction
   Syndrome 164
Postphlebitic Syndrome 164
Potter Facies 217
Potter Syndrome 164
Pott's Disease 69
Pott's Fracture 69
Pott's Puffy Tumour 70
Prader-Labhart-Willi
   Syndrome 165
Pringle's Disease 70
Prinzmetal's Angina 70
Prune Belly Syndrome 165

Pyle's Disease 70

Q Fever 70
Queckenstedt Test 218
Queensland Tick Typhus 71

Raeder's Syndrome 166
Ramsay-Hunt Syndrome 166
   (Herpes Zoster)
Ramsay-Hunt Syndrome 166
   (Cerebellar Ataxia)
Randall's Plaques 71
Rapunzel Syndrome 166
Raynaud's Disease 71
Raynaud's Phenomenon 72
Refsum's Syndrome 167
Reidel's Struma 72
Reinke's Oedema 72
Reiter's Disease 73
Remak Paralysis 73
Respiratory Distress
   Syndrome 167
Restless Legs Syndrome 167
Rett Syndrome 168
Reye's Syndrome 168
Richardson-Steele-
   Olszewski Syndrome 169
Rich's Focus 73
Richter's Hernia 74
Riddoch Syndrome 169
Rieger's Syndrome 169
Rift Valley Fever 74
Riley-Day Syndrome 169
Rinne Test 218
Ritter's Disease 74
Robin Hood Syndrome 170
Rockey's Sign 218
Rocky Mountain
   Spotted Fever 74

Medical Eponyms

Romana's Sign 218
Romberg's Sign 219
Rosai-Dorfman Disease 75
Ross River Fever 75
Rothmund's Syndrome 170
Roth's Spots 219
Rotor Syndrome 170
Roussy-Levy Syndrome 171
Rovsing's Sign 219
Rubinstein-Taybi Syndrome 171
Russell-Silver Syndrome 171
Russell Syndrome 171

Saegesser's Sign 219
Saint's Triad 219
Sandifer's Syndrome 172
Sanfilippo's Syndrome 172
Scalded Skin Syndrome 172
Scalenus Anticus Syndrome 172
Schatzki's Ring 75
Scheie's Syndrome 173
Scheuermann's Disease 76
Schilder's Disease 76
Schimmelbusch's Disease 76
Schlatter's Disease 77
Schmalz Test 220
Semiliki Forest Fever 77
Sever's Disease 77
Shakhonovich's Syndrome 173
Sheehan's Syndrome 173
Shenton's Line 220
Short Gut Syndrome 174
Shoulder-Hand Syndrome 174
Shy-Drager Syndrome 174
Sicca Syndrome 175
Sick Sinus Syndrome 175
Signe de Crochet 220
Signe de Dance 220
Silo-filler's Disease 77

Silver Syndrome 176
Simmond's Disease 77
Sindbis Fever 78
Singer's Nodes 78
Sipple's Syndrome 176
Sister Joseph's Nodule 220
Sjogren's Syndrome 176
Sjorgen-Larsson Syndrome 176
Sly Syndrome 177
Smith-Lemli-Opitz Syndrome 177
Smith's Fracture 78
Sotos Syndrome 177
Spiegler-Fendt Sarcoid 78
Spielmeyer-Vogt Disease 79
Spigelian Hernia 79
Spitz Naevus 79
Sprengel Deformity 79
St. Anthony's Fire 79
Stauffer's Syndrome 178
Steak House Syndrome 178
Steal Syndrome 178
Steinert's Disease 80
Stein-Leventhal Syndrome 178
Stellwag's Sign 220
Stevens-Johnson's Syndrome 178
Stewart Nasal Granuloma 80
Stickler Syndrome 179
Stiffman Syndrome 179
Still's Disease 80
St. Louis Fever 81
Stokes-Adams' Syndrome 179
Stuart-Treves Syndrome 180
Sturge-Weber Syndrome 180
St. Vitus Dance 81
Sudden Infant Death
    Syndrome 180
Sudek's Atrophy 81
Supermale Syndrome 181

Medical Eponyms

Sutton's Naevus 82
Sydenham's Chorea 82
Symes Amputation 82

Takayasu's Disease 82
Tangier Disease 83
Taravana Syndrome 181
Tarsal Tunnel Syndrome 181
Tay-Sachs Disease 83
Thomas Test 221
Thompson Test 221
Thomsen's Disease 84
Tietze's Syndrome 181
Tinel's Sign (Carpal
 Tunnel Syndrome) 221
Tinel's Sign
 (Nerve Regeneration) 221
Todd's Palsy 84
Tolosa Hunt Syndrome 182
Tourette's Syndrome 182
Toxic Shock Syndrome 182
Traube's Sign 221
Treacher-Collins Syndrome 183
Trendelenberg Sign 222
Trendelenberg Test 222
Trevor's Disease 84
Troisier's Sign 222
Trousseau's Sign (Tetany) 222
Trousseau's Sign
 (Thrombophlebitis) 223
Turcot's Syndrome 183
Turner's Syndrome 183

Uhthoff's Phenomenon 223
Urethral Syndrome 184
Usher's Syndrome 184

van Buchem Syndrome 184
van der Hoeve Syndrome 184

Verner-Morrison Syndrome 185
Vernet's Syndrome 185
Villaret's Syndrome 185
Vincent's Angina 85
Virchow Triad 85
Vogt-Koyanagi-Harada
 Syndrome 186
Volkmann's Contracture 85
von Gierke's Disease 85
von Graefe's Sign 223
von Hippel-Lindau Disease 86
von Recklinghausen's Disease 86
von Recklinghausen's
 Disease of Bone 87
von Willebrand's Disease 87

Waardenburg's Syndrome 186
Waldenstrom's
 Macroglobulinaemia 87
Wallenberg's Syndrome 186
Warthin's Tumour 88
Waterhouse-Friderichsen
 Syndrome 187
Weaver Syndrome 187
Weber's Syndrome 187
Weber Test 223
Wegener's Disease 88
Weill-Marchesani Syndrome 187
Weil's Disease 88
Werding-Hoffman Disease 89
Wermer's Syndrome 188
Werner's Syndrome 188
Wernicke-Korsakoff
 Syndrome 189
Wernicke's Aphasia 89
Wernicke's Encephalopathy 90
Westermark's Sign 224
West Nile Fever 90
West's Syndrome 189

Whipple's Disease 90
Wilkie's Disease 91
Williams Syndrome 189
Wilm's Tumour 91
Wilson's Disease 91
Wilson's Sign 224
Wiskott-Aldrich Syndrome 190
Wolff-Parkinson-White
   Syndrome 190
Wolf-Hirschorn Syndrome 191
Wool Sorter's Disease 92

Young's Syndrome 191

Zellweger Syndrome 191
Zollinger Ellison Syndrome 191
Zuelzer-Wilson Syndrome 192